Self-Assessment Colour Review of
Neuroimaging

Edited by

Kirsten Forbes
Institute of Neurological Sciences, Southern General Hospital, UK

Michael H. Lev
Director, Emergency Neuroradiology and Neurovascular Laboratory,
Massachusetts General Hospital, Boston, USA

Sanjay Shetty
Neuroradiology Section, Department of Radiology,
Massachusetts General Hospital, Boston, USA

Joseph Heiserman
Division of Neuroradiology, Barrow Neurological Institute,
St. Joseph's Hospital, Phoenix, USA

With contributions from

Jason Bearden
Division of Neuroradiology, Barrow Neurological Institute,
St. Joseph's Hospital, Phoenix, USA

Johannes B. Roedl
Department of Radiology, Massachusetts General Hospital, Boston, USA

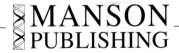

MANSON
PUBLISHING

Dedication

For Catriona, Eilidh, and Euan (KF)
For Greeshma and Sachin (SS)

Acknowledgement

To Jo Bhattacharya – who was involved in the initial concept and primary planning
of this book.

For full details of all Manson Publishing Ltd titles please write to:
Manson Publishing Ltd, 73 Corringham Road, London NW11 7DL, UK.
Tel: +44(0)20 8905 5150
Fax: +44(0)20 8201 9233
Email: manson@mansonpublishing.com
Website: www.mansonpublishing.com

Commissioning editor: Jill Northcott
Project manager: Paul Bennett
Copy editor: Ruth Maxwell
Layout: Cathy Martin, Presspack Computing Ltd
Colour reproduction: Tenon & Polert Colour Scanning Ltd, Hong Kong
Printed by: New Era Printing Company Ltd, Hong Kong

Preface

This concise volume is a case-based teaching text on imaging of the central nervous system. The book approaches neuroradiology in a practical day-to-day manner, offering readers over 100 real-life clinical cases for interpretation. It offers a visual, interactive mode of learning, designed to stimulate inquisitive thinking on a range of both common and more unusual neurological conditions.

While primarily written for radiologists, the wide range of cases will also be of interest to neurologists, neurosurgeons, and those many other physicians whose patients require imaging of the neuraxis, and who wish to learn more about neuroimaging.

The book is designed to simulate the clinical scenario: cases are presented with a short clinical history and a selection of pertinent images. A series of questions focuses the reader's mind on the important aspects of the case. The diagnosis is revealed on turning the page, whereby a discussion of not only imaging findings, but also differential diagnosis, pathology, and clinical correlation follow, and answers to the specific questions posed are indicated. Where imaging findings could be confused with alternate diagnoses, then these are shown, or readers are cross-referenced to other relevant parts of the text. Each case concludes with one or more 'take-home' teaching pearls.

This versatile book can be read in many ways: it may be used to test existing knowledge, which can then be enhanced by the supplementary information provided, or it can be used as a primary teaching text, whereby readers can select cases from the index. Regardless, the editors are hopeful that as you read it your interest in this fascinating subject will be (re)kindled and your knowledge of it will grow greater.

Kirsten Forbes
Michael Lev
Sanjay Shetty
Joseph Heiserman

3

Abbreviations

AC arachnoid cyst
ACA anterior cerebral artery
ACC agenesis of the corpus callosum
ACTH adrenocorticotrophic hormone
ADC apparent diffusion coefficient
ADEM acute disseminated encephalomyelitis
AED anti-epileptic drug
AHEM acute haemorrhagic encephalomyelitis
AIDS aquired immunodeficiency syndrome
(X-) ALD (X-linked) adrenoleukodystrophy
AML angiomyolipoma
AVM arteriovenous malformation
BDEM biphasic disseminated encephalomyelitis
BG brainstem glioma
CAA cerebral amyloid angiopathy
CADASIL cerebral autosomal dominant arteriopathy with subcortical infarct and leukoencephalopathy
CBV cerebral blood volume
CECT contrast enhanced computed tomography
CM cavernous malformation
CMV cytomegalovirus
CN cranial nerve
CNS central nervous system
CP craniopharyngioma
CPA cerebellopontine angle
CPP choroid plexus papilloma
CSF cerebrospinal fluid
CT computed tomography
CTA computed tomography angiography
CVT cortical venous thrombosis
DAI diffuse axonal injury
dAVF dural arteriovenous fistula
DNET dysembryoblastic neuroepithelial tumour
DS Devic's syndrome
DST dural sinus thrombosis
DTI diffusion tensor imaging
DWI diffusion weighted imaging

EBV Epstein–Barr virus
EDH epidural haematoma
EG eosinophilic granuloma
ESR erythrocyte sedimentation rate
FLAIR fluid inversion recovery
GBM glioblastoma multiforme
GC gliomatosis cerebri
GRE gradient recalled echo
HIV human immunodeficiency virus
HS Hallervorden–Spatz syndrome
HSE herpes simplex encephalitis
HSV herpes simplex virus
IAC internal auditory canal
ICA internal carotid artery/inferior cerebral artery
IPH intraparenchymal haematoma
JPA juvenile pilocytic astrocytoma
LCH Langerhans cell histiocytosis
LCM lymphocytic choriomeningitis
LHRH luteinizing hormone releasing hormone
MB medulloblastoma
MCA middle cerebral artery
MELAS mitochondrial myopathy, encephalopathy, lactic acidosis and stroke-like episodes
MIP maximum intensity projection
MISME multiple inherited schwannomas, meningiomas, and ependymomas
MLD metachromatic leukodystrophy
MRA magnetic resonance angiography
MRI magnetic resonance imaging
MRS magnetic resonance spectroscopy
MRV magnetic resonance venography
MS multiple sclerosis
MTS mesial temporal sclerosis
MVA motor vehicle accident
NAA n-acetyl aspartate
NECT nonenhanced computed tomography
NF 1,2 neurofibromatosis type 1,2
NPH normal pressure hydrocephalus
NSAID nonsteroidal anti-inflammatory drugs

PCA posterior cerebral artery
PCNSL primary CNS lymphoma
PKAN pantothenate kinase-associated
   neurodegeneration
PML progressive multifocal
   leukoencephalopathy
PNET primitive neuroectodermal tumour
PPP pseudophlebitic pattern
PRES posterior reversible
   encephalopathy syndrome
PXA pleomorphic xanthoastrocytoma
RA rheumatoid arthritis
RLVD retrograde leptomeningeal venous
   drainage
SDE subdural empyema
SDH subdural haematoma
SIADH syndrome of inappropriate
   antidiuretic hormone

SLE systemic lupus erythematosus
SNHL sensorineural hearing loss
SOD septo-optic dysplasia
S-PNET supratentorial primitive
   neuroectodermal tumour
STIR short tau inversion recovery
TB tuberculosis
TBI traumatic brain injury
TIA transient ischaemic attack
TOF time-of-flight
TORCH (t)oxoplasmosis, (o)ther,
   (r)ubella, (c)ytomegalovirus, (h)erpes
   simplex
TSC tuberous sclerosis complex
VHL von Hippel–Lindau syndrome
WBC white blood cell
WHO World Health Organization
WM white matter

Classification of cases

Abscess, epidural: 106
Abscess, pyogenic: 83
Acoustic schwannoma: 62
Acute disseminated encephalomyelitis:
   90
Adrenoleukodystrophy: 19
Agenesis of corpus callosum: 1
Alobar holoprosencephaly: 7
Aneurysm, anterior communicating: 25
   middle cerebral artery: 81
Anti-epileptic drug-related white matter
   changes: 29
Arachnoiditis: 97
Arteriovenous malformation: 32
CADASIL: 58
Cavernous malformation: 52
Cerebral amyloid angiopathy: 71
Chondrosarcoma: 91
Choroid plexus carcinoma: 108
Choroid plexus papilloma: 102
Cord degeneration: 26

Craniopharyngioma: 96
Cyst, arachnoid: 31
   dermoid: 42
   epidermoid: 8
   facet joint: 48
   pineal: 59
Cytomegalovirus, congenital: 51
Dandy–Walker malformation: 23
Developmental delay:
   rhomboencephalosynapsis: 14
   septo-optic dysplasia: 82
Devic's syndrome: 9
Diffuse axonal injury: 73
Disc herniation, right C6/7: 15
Dural arteriovenous fistula: 11
Dysembryoblastic neuroepithelial
   tumour: 5
Ependymoma: 109
Epidural haematoma: 45, 63
Epidural lipomatosis 60
Extracranial ICA dissection: 46

5

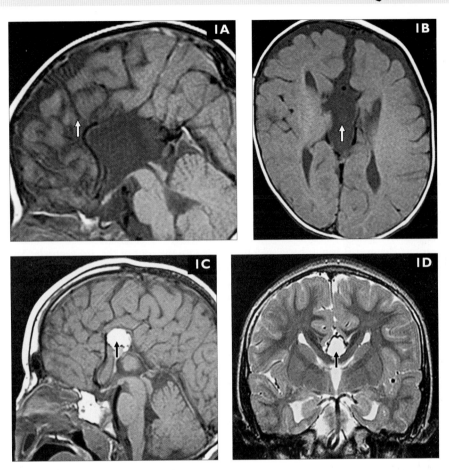

1 A 6-month old child presents with seizures.
i. Describe the features shown on imaging (**1A, B**).
ii. What is the diagnosis?
iii. What are its associations?
iv. How does the companion case shown (**1C, D**) differ?

I: Answer

1 DIAGNOSIS Agenesis of the corpus callosum (**ii**).

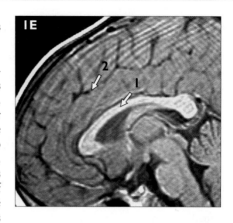

IMAGING FINDINGS The sagittal T1-weighted MRI image (**1A**) reveals agenesis of the corpus callosum (ACC). This is the largest white matter commissure in the brain, lying in the midline, where it connects the two cerebral hemispheres (**1E**, arrow 1). Normal development of the corpus callosum is associated with inversion of the cingulate gyrus forming the cingulate sulcus, which parallels the corpus callosum superiorly (**1E**, arrow 2). Thus, in ACC, the cingulate sulcus is absent, causing the medial hemispheric sulci to radiate into the roof of the 3rd ventricle (**1A**, arrow). The axial T1-weighted MRI (**1B**), reveals the resultant high-riding 3rd ventricle extending superiorly between parallel lateral ventricles (arrow). The trigones and occipital horns of the lateral ventricles are often dilated in ACC, termed colpocephaly (**i**).

PATHOLOGY AND CLINICAL CORRELATION The corpus callosum forms during the first trimester and its absence (agenesis) or incomplete formation (hypogenesis) may result from one of many different genetic mutations. Associated developmental anomalies are common and include Chiari II malformation, Dandy–Walker malformation, and disorders of neuronal migration and organization. ACC is also a feature of many different syndromes, for example Aicardi syndrome. In this X-linked syndrome, ACC is associated with an interhemispheric cyst, cortical dysplasia (commonly polymicrogyria), grey matter heterotopia, and hypoplasic cerebellum (**iii**).

COMPANION CASE

DIAGNOSIS Hypogenesis of the corpus callosum with interhemispheric lipoma.

IMAGING FINDINGS The sagittal T1-weighted MRI image (**1C**) shows that only part of the corpus callosum has formed (anterior body). The posterior body, splenium, and rostrum of the corpus callosum are absent. On both the T1-weighted image and the coronal T2-weighted image (**1D**), a focal hyperintense mass is seen in the midline, posterior and superior to the formed corpus callosum (arrow). This is an interhemispheric lipoma, which is almost always associated with agenesis or hypogenesis of the corpus callosum.

Pathology and clinical correlation The corpus callosum develops in an orderly fashion starting with posterior genu, body, anterior genu, splenium, and lastly rostrum. Knowledge of this normal pattern of development makes it is possible to differentiate a hypogenetic corpus callosum from one that has been secondarily damaged. Interhemispheric lipoma develops from abnormal differentiation of the mesenchyme that surrounds the developing brain (meninx primitiva).

Teaching pearl
➤ *Agenesis of the corpus callosum is commonly associated with other intracranial developmental anomalies.*

Reference
Barkovich AJ, Norman D (1988). Anomalies of the corpus callosum: correlation with further anomalies of the brain. *AJNR* 9:493–501.

---

2 A 20-year-old female patient presents with decreased vision in her left eye.
i. Define the abnormal structure in image 2A.
ii. Is extraocular muscle enhancement normal?
iii. Is the optic nerve encased by Schwann cells or meninges?

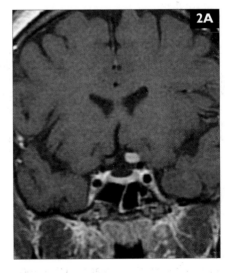

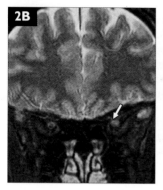

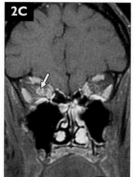

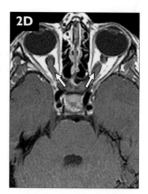

2 **DIAGNOSIS** Optic neuritis.

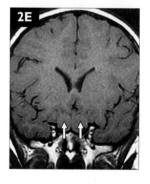

IMAGING FINDINGS Coronal T2 image (**2B**) shows subtle diffuse increased signal throughout the substance of the left optic nerve. Postcontrast T1 image (**2A**) reveals corresponding diffuse enhancement and confirms enlargement of the nerve (**i**). No perineural mass is present. The right optic nerve appears normal. Note that the extraocular muscles normally enhance (**ii**).

Companion cases (different patients) demonstrate perineural enhancement on postcontrast T1 coronal image in **2C** in a patient with an optic nerve meningioma. Images **2D** and **2E** are nice examples of severe bilateral nodular optic nerve enlargement due to bilateral optic nerve gliomas.

DIFFERENTIAL DIAGNOSIS The primary consideration when enhancement is noted related to the optic nerve is differentiation between enhancement of the actual nerve and enhancement of the adjacent meningeal lining (optic nerves are lined by meninges rather than schwann cells seen with peripheral nerves [**iii**]). In this case (**2A, B**), the nerve itself is clearly involved.

When nerve enhancement is present, the next determination is whether or not there is mass-like enlargement to suggest optic glioma. This case demonstrates only minimal diffuse enlargement and associated oedema (T2 hyperintensity). The primary differential considerations are optic neuritis or optic nerve vasculitis (most commonly related to infection, radiation, or autoimmune disorders). Optic neuritis is much more common and is the correct diagnosis in this case.

PATHOLOGY AND CLINICAL CORRELATION Though postcontrast fat saturation sequences show a 95% sensitivity in identifying optic nerve enhancement, MRI is not necessary for diagnosis of optic neuritis in the majority of cases. Occasionally, patients with nonarteritic anterior ischaemic optic neuropathy, acute compressive neuropathy secondary to a pituitary tumour or aneurysm, or posterior scleritis have symptoms mimicking optic neuritis and MRI provides the correct diagnosis. More commonly, the diagnosis of optic neuritis is known and the clinical question is whether or not the neuritis is an isolated finding. There is a strong association between optic neuritis and multiple sclerosis (MS). Indeed, approximately 20% of MS patients initially present with optic neuritis. Furthermore, 50–60% of patients with optic neuritis will be diagnosed with MS over the subsequent 15 years.

Interestingly, the length of nerve enhancement with optic neuritis appears to correlate with initial severity of visual impairment (both colour perception and special resolution). However, there is no correlation between degree of enhancement and final recovery of function. Steroids are administered as the mainstay of treatment and the patients are followed closely for the development of MS.

TEACHING PEARLS
➢ *Postcontrast fat saturation T1 images are highly sensitive for the detection of optic nerve enhancement.*
➢ *50–60% of patients with optic neuritis progress to MS.*
➢ *20% of patients with MS present with optic neuritis.*

REFERENCES
Frith JA, McLeod JG, Hely M (2000). Acute optic neuritis in Australia: a 13 year prospective study. *J Neurol Neurosurg Psychiatry* **68**:246–56.
Kupersmith MJ, *et al.* (2002). Contrast-enhanced MRI in acute optic neuritis: relationship to visual performance. *Brain* **125**:812–22.
Sorensen TL, *et al.* (1999). Optic neuritis as onset manifestation of multiple sclerosis: a nationwide, long-term survey. *Neurology* **53**(3):473–8.

3 A 30-year-old male patient presents with complex partial seizures.
i. Name structures 1–3 on this coronal T2-weighted 3T MR (3).
ii. What are the imaging findings?
iii. What is the diagnosis?

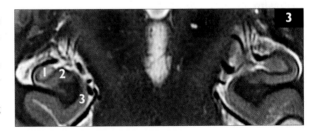

3 **DIAGNOSIS** Right mesial temporal sclerosis (MTS) (iii).

IMAGING FINDINGS Structure 1: CA4/dentate; structure 2: subiculum; structure 3: parahippocampal gyrus (i). The right hippocampus is both shrunken and hyperintense on T2-weighted imaging (ii). This affects all parts of the hippocampal body shown, the CA1–4 areas of the cornu ammonis (see below). Other associated findings included loss of hippocampal structure and hippocampal head digitations, dilatation of the ipsilateral temporal horn of the lateral ventricle, local white matter changes, as well as atrophy of the fornix and mamillary bodies.

DIFFERENTIAL DIAGNOSIS The presence of T2 hyperintensity in a shrunken hippocampus is pathognomonic of mesial temporal sclerosis. However, if a T2 hyperintense hippocampus is enlarged, then tumour, infection (herpes simplex encephalitis), and post-seizure appearance should be considered.

PATHOLOGY AND CLINICAL CORRELATION MTS is found in some patients with temporal lobe complex partial seizures and is the most common cause for epilepsy surgery. Histological examination reveals pyramidal and granule cell neuronal loss in the cornu ammonis and dentate sections of the hippocampus. The cornu ammonis can be further subdivided into 4 areas CA1–CA4. Medially, it blends into the subiculum and then onto the parahippocampal gyrus.

There is some debate over whether MTS is an acquired or developmental pathology. Temporal imaging changes showing the development of MTS have been well-documented following prolonged seizures, supporting an acquired pathophysiology. However, it has also been observed that MTS is associated with a second developmental abnormality (dual pathology) in 15% of cases.

TEACHING PEARLS
➣ *The imaging findings of MTS are a shrunken, T2 hyperintense hippocampus.*
➣ *Underlying pathophysiology is still debated.*

REFERENCE
Duvernoy HM, *et al.* (1988). *The Human Hippocampus: Functional Anatomy, Vascularization, and Serial Sections with MRI*, 3rd edn. Springer Verlag, Berlin.

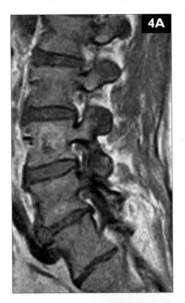
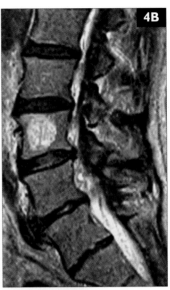

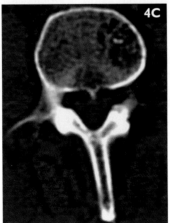

4 A patient presents with low back pain, and the following images are obtained (4A–C).

i. Define the level of the vertebral abnormality.

ii. What is the significance of intrinsic increased T1 signal?

iii. What is the name given to the CT appearance in 4C?

4 DIAGNOSIS Vertebral haemangioma.

IMAGING FINDINGS This case demonstrates the classic appearance of vertebral haemangiomas on MRI and CT. There is a mass within the left aspect of the L3 vertebral body showing increased T1 (**4A**) and T2 (**4B**) signal (**i**). CT demonstrates the characteristic 'polka-dot' appearance of the lesion due to axial cuts through thickened vertical trabeculae (**4C**) (**iii**). The degree of T1 hyperintensity is variable and correlates with the degree of fatty stroma within the mass (**ii**). Haemangiomas with more fat/T1 hyperintensity are considered less likely to evolve into larger or clinically significant lesions. Though not demonstrated in this case, radiographs of the spine would show coarse vertical striations or a 'honeycomb' appearance. Rarely, osseous lesions will have a soft tissue component that may show vascular flow voids on MRI.

DIFFERENTIAL DIAGNOSIS The differential diagnosis of a vertebral body lesion consists of metastatic disease and primary tumours of bone. The classic T1 and T2 hyperintensity on MRI and the 'polka-dot' CT appearance when present are essentially pathognomonic of vertebral haemangioma.

PATHOLOGY AND CLINICAL CORRELATION Vertebral haemangiomas are common lesions occurring in up to 10% of the population. They are almost always confined to the vertebral body and do not involve the posterior elements. These masses are most commonly clinically silent and only found incidentally. Rarely, they can be a source of focal back pain and can occasionally cause spinal cord or nerve root compression due to osseous or soft tissue tumour expansion, associated epidural haematoma, or compression fracture.

In general, asymptomatic haemangiomas require no dedicated follow-up unless they become painful. Lesions that are painful at presentation but do not cause cord compression or radicular symptoms should be followed by annual clinical and radiographic exams. As noted above, fat content is associated with nonevolving lesions. Conversely, lesions with little or no fat/T1 hyperintensity are more likely to undergo evolution/growth. Haemangioma growth has been associated with late stages of pregnancy, presumably due to physiologic vascular and haemodynamic changes.

Treatment for symptomatic lesions involves surgical decompression when necessary to relieve compressive symptoms. Focal radiation, embolization, and/or vertebroplasty are used to treat lesions associated with refractory pain only.

TEACHING PEARLS
➤ *Vertebral haemangiomas are common lesions and are most often incidental findings in patients with no symptoms or with pain due to another cause.*
➤ *Occasionally, vertebral haemangiomas can show aggressive features and growth. This can be a source of pain and/or spinal or nerve root compression.*
➤ *Follow-up imaging is not required for clinically silent haemangiomas that show classic imaging features.*

REFERENCES (CASE 4)

Fox MW, Onofrio BM (1993). The natural history and management of symptomatic and asymptomatic vertebral haemangiomas. *J Neurosurg* **78**:36–45.

Tekkok IH, *et al.* (1993). Vertebral haemangioma symptomatic during pregnancy – Report of a case and review of the literature. *Neurosurgery* **32**(2):302–6.

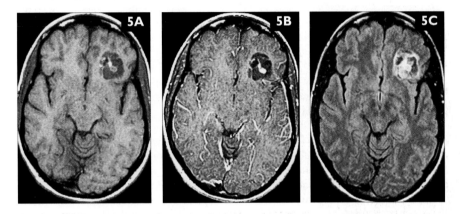

5 A 16-year-old female patient presents with a history of long-standing partial complex seizures, and the following images are obtained (**5A–C**).

i. Which sequences are shown?

ii. Where is the lesion located?

iii. What is the differential diagnosis, given the patient's history?

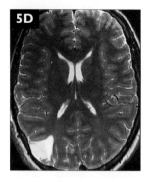

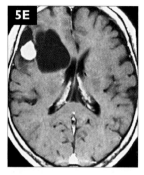

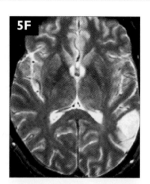

5 DIAGNOSIS Dysembryoblastic neuroepithelial tumour (DNET).

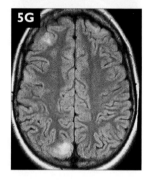

IMAGING FINDINGS Images 5A–C (axial T1, axial postcontrast T1, and axial FLAIR, respectively) demonstrate a nonenhancing, pseudocystic, multinodular mass in the white matter of the left frontal lobe (**i, ii**). The lesion is predominantly T1 hypointense and appears heterogenous on the FLAIR sequence with a surrounding hyperintense rim. The tumour is well demarcated and is not associated with oedema or mass effect. Image **5D** shows a T2-weighted image of another case of DNET with typical features: a hyperintense, pseudocystic, intracortical wedge-shaped mass pointing towards the ventricle.

DIFFERENTIAL DIAGNOSIS The differential diagnosis (**iii**) of a peripherally located supratentorial mass in a child or young adult presenting with seizure includes:
- DNET.
- Low-grade astrocytoma (**5F**, axial T2).
- Ganglioglioma.
- Oligodendroglioma.
- Pleomorphic xanthoastrocytoma
- Pleomorphic xanthoastrocytoma (PXA) (**5E**, axial postcontrast T1)
- Tubers in tuberous sclerosis (TSC) (**5G**, FLAIR)
- Neurocysticercosis.

The usual appearance of DNET is a homogeneously T2 hyperintense cortical lesion, so the major differential possibility in the usual setting would be a low-grade astrocytoma. Low-grade astrocytoma (**5F**) resembles the more typical T2 hyperintense wedge-shaped appearance of the DNET in 5D; like DNETs, low-grade astrocytomas typically do not enhance. Other less likely possibilities for a cortical T2 hyperintense lesion would include infarct or demyelination.

Lesions with a more heterogeneous or cystic/nodular appearance would be less likely to be confused with a DNET, except when the lesion has a more unusual appearance, as in this case. Image 5E depicts the typical morphology of a PXA with a mural nodule at the margin of a large cyst in a patient with long-standing epilepsy.

Cortical/subcortical tubers in TSC (**5G**) are usually multifocal and associated with other features of TSC, including subependymal nodules.

PATHOLOGY AND CLINICAL CORRELATION DNETs are benign, mostly cortical masses superimposed on cortical dysplasia with the majority involving the temporal lobe. DNETs are typically identified before age 20 years in patients with long-standing partial complex seizures. Some authors assert that they are the most common structural lesions in children with partial seizures. Showing no or very slow growth and rare recurrence after surgical resection, DNETs are classified as grade 1 tumours by the WHO.

TEACHING PEARLS
➢ *DNETs occur in children or young adults with long-standing partial complex seizures.*
➢ *DNETs are benign, T2 hyperintense, multinodular, well-demarcated, wedge-shaped intracortical masses.*

REFERENCES
Osborn AG, *et al.* (2004). *Brain*. Amirsys, Salt Lake City, Chapter I-6, pp.66–9, 76–9.
Selch MT, *et al.* (1998). Gangliogliomas: experience with 34 patients and review of the literature. *Am J Clin Oncol* 21(6):557–64.
Stanescu Cosson R, *et al.* (2001). Dysembryoblastic neuroepithelial tumours: CT, MR findings and imaging follow-up: a study of 53 cases. *J Neuroradiol* 28(4):230–40.

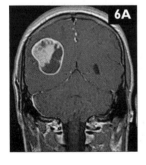 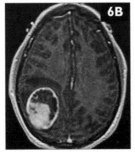 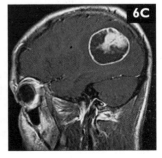

6 A 16-year-old child presents with weakness and the following images are obtained (6A–C)
i. What lobe is the mass centred within?
ii. What is the extent of surrounding oedema?
iii. Name several classic cerebral lesions associated with a cyst and mural nodule.

6 **DIAGNOSIS** Pleomorphic xanthoastrocytoma.

IMAGING FINDINGS A large mass is seen centred within the right parietal lobe (i) on postcontrast T1 coronal, axial, and sagittal images (**6A, 6B,** and **6C** respectively). The mass is composed of a nonenhancing cyst and a diffusely enhancing mural nodule. There is relatively mild surrounding oedema (ii). The axial image shows tumour extension to the brain periphery. No other lesions are present. Though not presented, the mass is hypoattenuating on CT and shows intrinsic T1 hypointensity and T2 hyperintensity on nonenhanced MR images.

DIFFERENTIAL DIAGNOSIS Imaging findings are nonspecific. Classic primary CNS tumours that can demonstrate a cyst and mural nodule configuration are haemangioblastoma, juvenile pilocytic astrocytoma (JPA), and pleomorphic xanthoastrocytoma (PXA) (iii). However, additional primary and metastatic tumours would be considered in this case.

As the name implies, PXAs are histologically pleomorphic. Not surprisingly, imaging findings are variable. The classic appearance is that of a cystic supratentorial mass containing an avidly enhancing mural nodule that is adjacent to the peripheral leptomeninges (as in this case). It is the peripheral location that is the most consistent imaging finding. Surrounding oedema is usually modest relative to the size of the mass.

PATHOLOGY AND CLINICAL CORRELATION PXAs are rare primary brain neoplasms accounting for less than 1% of all brain tumours. Nonetheless, familiarity with this entity is important as they are highly amenable to surgical extirpation. Indeed, postresection survival is reported as 81% at 5 years and 70% at 10 years. Recurrent disease, when present, is also treated with surgery as the tumours are generally unresponsive to chemotherapy or radiation.

PXAs can occur in any age group but are most often encountered in adolescents or young adults. A long history of seizure is the most common presenting complaint. Almost all are supratentorial, most commonly within the temporal (49%) or parietal lobes (17%). Though commonly attached to the meninges, actual invasion of the dura is rare.

TEACHING PEARLS
➤ *PXAs are rare tumours that are most commonly seen in a supratentorial peripheral location abutting the meninges.*
➤ *A cyst and mural nodule is the most common appearance but is seen in only 50% of cases.*
➤ *PXAs are treated with surgical resection, which can be curative.*

REFERENCES (CASE 6)

Giannini C, *et al*. (1999). Pleomorphic xanthoastrocytoma: what do we really know about it? *Cancer* **85**:2033–45.

Koeller KK, Henry JM (2001). Superficial gliomas: radiologic-pathologic correlation. *Radiographics* **21**:1533–56.

Pahapill PA, Ramsay DA, Del Maestro RF (1996). Pleomorphic xanthoastrocytoma: case report and analysis of the literature concerning the efficacy of resection and the significance of necrosis. *Neurosurgery* **38**:822–9.

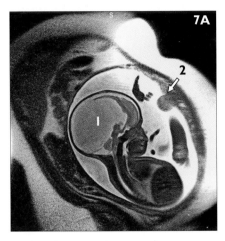

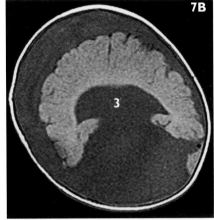

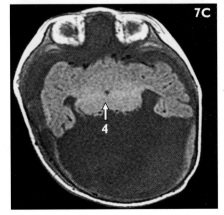

7 A pregnant female presents with macrocephaly on detailed fetal ultrasound.

i. Describe the features shown on prenatal MR imaging (**7A**).

ii. What is the differential diagnosis?

iii. Does postnatal MRI (**7B, C**) help in the diagnosis?

7: Answer

7 **DIAGNOSIS** Alobar holoprosencephaly.

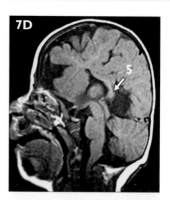

IMAGING FINDINGS The prenatal MRI obtained in the sagittal plane (**7A**) shows a large cerebrospinal fluid (CSF) filled space within the posterior aspect of the supratentorial cranium (**1**). A thin layer of cortex is present anteriorly (arrow **2**), but brain parenchyma can not be distinguished posteriorly. The corpus callosum is not present (**i**). Postnatal axial T1-weighted MRI (**7B, C**) shows a central monoventricle extending into a dorsal cyst (**3**). The 3rd ventricle is absent, due to fusion of the thalami (arrow **4**). Rudimentary temporal horns are the only remnant of the lateral ventricles. The brain parenchyma comprises a 'pancake-like' mass of tissue seen in the anterior cranium, with a prominent anterior subarachnoid space. There is absence of the interhemispheric fissure, falx cerebri, and corpus callosum (**iii**).

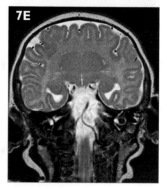

DIFFERENTIAL DIAGNOSIS Differential diagnosis includes holoprosencephaly, hydranencephaly, and maximal hydrocephlus (**ii**).

PATHOLOGY AND CLINICAL CORRELATION Holoprosencephaly results from a failure of the forebrain to divide completely into two separate cerebral hemispheres. These remain fused to varying degrees leading to a continuum of abnormalities, termed alobar (most severe), semilobar, and lobar (mildest) holoprosencephaly.

This malformation may result from both teratogenic influences, e.g. material diabetes or genetic factors. Presentation depends on the severity of the forebrain fusion and varies from epilepsy or develomental delay to stillbirth or early neonatal mortality. Patients with alobar holoprosencephaly commonly have midline facial anomalies, most severely cyclopia (fusion of the orbits).

The less severe case of holoprosencephaly (semilobar) shown (**7D, E**) shows partial cleavage of the hemispheres with formation of the posterior body and splenium of corpus callosum (arrow **5**) and development of the posterior interhemispheric fissure. The rostral brain remain fused.

TEACHING PEARL

 Holoprosencephaly occurs when the cerebral hemispheres fail to separate.

REFERENCE

Simon EM, Barkovich AJ (2001). Holoprosencephaly: new concepts. *Magn Reson Imaging Clin N Am* 9(1):149–64, viii–ix.

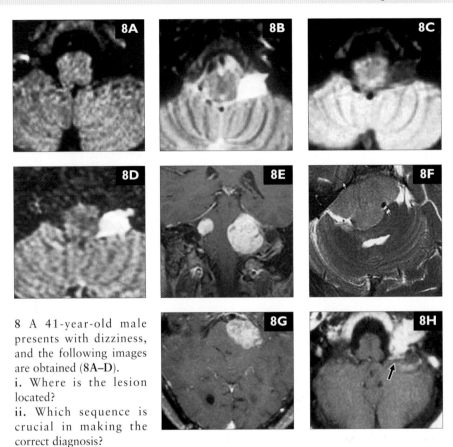

8 A 41-year-old male presents with dizziness, and the following images are obtained (8A–D).
i. Where is the lesion located?
ii. Which sequence is crucial in making the correct diagnosis?

DIFFERENTIAL DIAGNOSIS Images 8E–H.

8 **DIAGNOSIS** Epidermoid cyst.

IMAGING FINDINGS Images 8A–D (axial T1, axial T2, axial FLAIR, DWI, respectively) demonstrate a T2 hyperintense cystic mass in the left cerebellopontine angle (CPA) (i), that does not enhance and does not completely attenuate in the FLAIR sequence. Restricted diffusion seen on DWI clinches the diagnosis (ii).

DIFFERENTIAL DIAGNOSIS The differential diagnosis of a CPA mass includes:
Solid:
• Vestibular schwannoma (8E, coronal contrast-enhanced T1).
• Meningioma (8F, axial T2).
• Metastasis (8G, axial contrast-enhanced T1).
• Lipoma.
Cyst-like:
• Epidermoid cyst (8A–D).
• Arachnoid cyst (see Question 31).
Other:
• Jugular foramen paraganglioma (8H, axial contrast-enhanced T1).
The 'big four' in the CPA are vestibular schwannoma, meningioma, epidermoid cyst, and arachnoid cyst. In reality, one can narrow the differential possibilities rapidly based on even a cursory glance at the lesion. Lesions that resemble cerebrospinal fluid include arachnoid cyst and epidermoid, while meningioma and schwannoma are solid, homogeneously enhancing lesions.

Image 8E demonstrates avidly enhancing well-circumscribed vestibular schwannomas in the CPAs bilaterally, in a patient with neurofibromatosis type 2 (NF2). The typical appearance of a large dural-based T2 isointense meningioma centred along the posterior petrous wall is shown in image 8F. Schwannomas are T2 hyperintense and often expand the porus acusticus. A nodular heterogenous enhancing mass in the left CPA represents a metastasis from primary lung cancer (8G).

The jugular foramen paraganglioma in 8H is characterized as an intense contrast enhancing lesion that has expanded the jugular foramen and extends medially into the CPA cistern (arrow); note how this lesion is centred outside of the CPA in the region of the jugular foramen, opening up an entirely different list of considerations.

PATHOLOGY AND CLINICAL CORRELATION An epidermoid cyst is a congenital intradural lesion arising from inclusion of ectodermal epithelial elements during neural tube closure. This 3rd most common CPA mass is a congenital slow-growing lesion that remains silent for many years with a peak age of 40 years. Although total surgical removal is possible only in less than 50% of cases, the outcome is good, because growth is slow in case of recurrence. Restricted diffusion, manifested as increased signal on DWI, is the imaging hallmark of epidermoids.

TEACHING PEARLS

➤ *Epidermoid cyst is the 3rd most common CPA mass after vestibular schwannoma and meningioma.*
➤ *High signal on DWI and incomplete attenuation on FLAIR is diagnostic and helps to distinguish the lesion from arachnoid cyst.*
➤ *Cystic lesions (epidermoid and arachnoid) are easily distinguished from solid lesions of the CPA.*
➤ *Diffusion can also be used to diagnose recurrent epidermoid.*
➤ *75% of epidermoids occur in the CPA, 25% in the 4th ventricle.*

REFERENCE

Dutt SN, *et al.* (2002). Radiologic differentiation of intracranial epidermoids from arachnoid cysts. *Otol Neurotol* **23**:84–92.

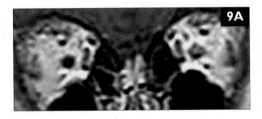

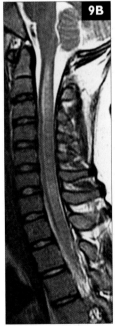

9 A 14-year-old child presents with suspected optic neuritis. The following images are obtained (**9A, B**).
i. What structure is abnormal in the first image?
ii. Is the abnormality unilateral or bilateral?
iii. What is a differential diagnosis for isolated intramedullary cord signal abnormality?

9 DIAGNOSIS Devic's syndrome (DS), neuromyelitis optica.

IMAGING FINDINGS Coronal postcontrast T1 image (**9A**) through the posterior orbits shows enhancement and mild enlargement of the left optic nerve (**i**). The right optic nerve appears normal (**ii**). Sagittal T2 image of the cervical spine in the same patient several months later demonstrates intramedullary T2 hyperintensity and cord expansion extending from C1 to at least T2 (**9B**).

DIFFERENTIAL DIAGNOSIS It is sometimes difficult to determine if enhancement relates to the optic nerve itself or the meningeal lining of the nerve. However, when nerve enhancement and expansion are clearly identified (as in this case), optic neuritis is most common. Optic gliomas also enhance and expand the nerve, but are more commonly focal and demonstrate a more gradual clinical onset.

Intramedullary cord signal abnormality and expansion raise concern for neoplasm, focal myelitis ('transverse myelitis'), multiple sclerosis (MS) and, rarely, infection (**iii**).

PATHOLOGY AND CLINICAL CORRELATION Devic's syndrome is an inflammatory demyelinating disease characterized by attacks of optic neuritis (uni- or bilateral) and focal myelitis with sparing of the brain itself. Diagnosis requires both index events though they may or may not present simultaneously. There are both monophasic and relapsing forms of the disease. Patients with the monophasic form generally present with more severe symptoms but relapsing patients show worse long-term function. Long-term follow-up studies have shown functional blindness in at least one eye in over half of the patients with relapsing form, and approximately 25% of those with monophasic disease. Similarly, permanent monoplegia or paraplegia was found in approximately 50% of the relapsing group and 30% of the monophasic group.

The aetiology of DS is controversial but evidence tends to point toward a distinct entity rather than a variant of MS. First, imaging characteristics are different. While both are associated with optic neuritis, DS spares the brain. Additionally, spinal lesions in DS are much larger than those in MS, generally spanning three or more vertebral segments. Second, the clinical severity of DS differs from MS. As noted above, long-term deficits can be quite severe in DS. With relapsing disease especially, respiratory failure is a significant concern, occurring in up to 1/3 of patients (and resulting in death in 93% of those affected in one retrospective study).

TEACHING PEARLS
- *DS is an inflammatory demyelinating disease causing optic neuritis and focal myelopathy.*
- *There are both monophasic and relapsing forms of the disease but both appear to be distinct entities rather than a form of MS.*
- *Long-term deficits can be severe.*

REFERENCES (CASE 9)

Filippi M, *et al.* (1999). MRI and magnetization transfer imaging changes in the brain and cervical cord of patients with Devic's neuromyelitis optica. *Neurology* 53(8):1705–10.

Lucchinetti CF, *et al.* (2002). A role for humoral mechanisms in the pathogenesis of Devic's neuromyelitis optica. *Brain* 125(7):1450–61.

Wingerchuk DM, *et al.* (1999). The clinical course of neuromyelitis optica (Devic's syndrome). *Neurology* 53(5):1107–14.

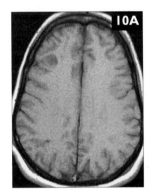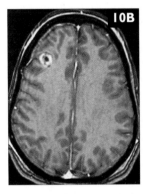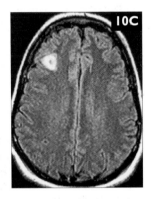

10 A 17-year-old female presents with intermittent partial complex seizures. The following images are obtained (**10A–C**).

i. Which sequences are shown and what are the imaging findings?

ii. What is the differential diagnosis?

10 DIAGNOSIS Ganglioglioma

IMAGING FINDINGS Images 10A–C (axial T1, axial postcontrast T1, and axial FLAIR, respectively) (i) reveal a ring enhancing lesion in the subcortical white matter of the right frontal lobe (ii) which is hypointense on T1 and peripherally hyperintense on FLAIR.

DIFFERENTIAL DIAGNOSIS The differential diagnosis (iii) of this lesion includes:
- Pleomorphic xanthoastrocytoma (5E).
- Oligodengroglioma.
- Dysembryoplastic neuroepithelial tumour (DNET) (5A–C).
- Pilocytic astrocytoma.
- Neurocysticercosis.
- Low-grade astrocytoma.

Gangliogliomas can be either cystic appearing with a mural nodule (classic description), solid, or infiltrating (rare). They are most commonly located in the superficial hemispheres or temporal lobes in a cortical/subcortical location. Heterogeneous enhancement and calcification are common. See Question 5 for a discussion of other entities in the differential diagnosis.

PATHOLOGY AND CLINICAL CORRELATION Gangliogliomas are well-differentiated tumours (WHO Grade 1 or 2) composed of glial and ganglion cells. They can be associated with cortical dysplasia. The diagnosis should be considered in a young patient (80% occur in patient under 30 years of age, with a peak incidence between 10–20 years) with a cortically based cystic appearing or solid lesion. Calcification is common (up to 50%) as is heterogeneous enhancement. The tumour is the most common cause of chronic temporal lobe epilepsy. Other presenting symptoms, such as headaches, can be related to mass effect. Clinical prognosis is excellent following complete resection, including resolution of seizures in the majority of patients (80%). Higher grade lesions are uncommon (5–10%).

TEACHING PEARLS
➤ *A partially cystic, enhancing mass with a mural nodule in the superficial hemispheres or temporal lobes is classic, but nonspecific for ganglioglioma.*
➤ *Ganglioglioma occur in children or young adults.*
➤ *Ganglioglioma is the most common neoplasm causing chronic temporal lobe epilepsy.*
➤ *80% of patients are seizure-free after surgical resection of ganglioglioma.*
➤ *Patient age peak incidence is 10–20 years.*

REFERENCES
Osborn AG, *et al.* (2004). Brain. Amirsys, Salt Lake City, Chapter I-6, pp. 66–9, 76–9.
Selch MT, *et al.* (1998). Gangliogliomas: experience with 34 patients and review of the literature. *Am J Clin Oncol* **21**(6):557–64.

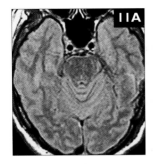

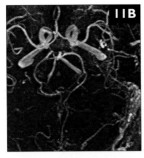

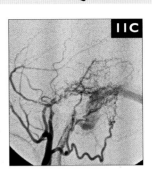

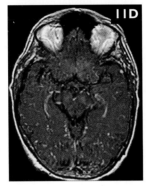

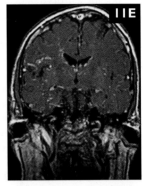

11 A 42-year-old patient presents with pulsatile tinnitus. The following images are obtained (11A–C). Images 11D–F are from a 65-year-old patient with rapidly progressing dementia.

i. What artery was injected for the angiogram in 11C?

ii. What is the name given to the imaging finding in images 11D and E?

iii. Name several causes of pulsatile tinnitus.

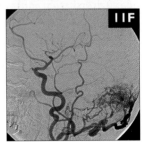

11 DIAGNOSIS Dural arteriovenous fistula (dAVF).

IMAGING FINDINGS Axial proton density image (**11A**) demonstrates the subtle finding of multiple small vascular flow voids adjacent to the junction of the left transverse and sigmoid sinuses. Additionally, a small focus of hyperintense signal is seen within the adjacent left temporal lobe. MRA volumetric image (**11B**) confirms multiple abnormal vessels adjacent to the left transverse and sigmoid sinuses. Digital subtraction angiography from a left external carotid injection confirms the diagnosis by clearly showing multiple enlarged feeding arteries converging on the adjacent dural sinuses (**i**). Note filling of the sinus while still in the arterial phase of injection.

Companion case images show an unusual pattern of diffusely enlarged cortical veins on postcontrast axial and coronal T1 images (**11D, E**). The term pseudophlebitic pattern (PPP) has been used to describe this finding (**ii**). As in the first case, digital subtraction angiography of the external carotid artery confirms shunting between the arterial supply and the dural venous sinuses.

DIFFERENTIAL DIAGNOSIS Clinical differential diagnosis for objective (physician confirmed) pulsatile tinnitus is quite extensive. The most common causes include serous otitis media, high riding jugular bulb, glomus tympanicum, systemic disorders of high cardiac output (anemia, thyrotoxicosis), arteriovenous malformation (AVM), dAVF, and arterial wall disorders such as dissection, atherosclerosis, or aneurysm (**iii**).

When arteriovenous shunting is demonstrated, the primary differential is between pial AVM, mixed pial/dural AVM, and dAVF. Angiogram should be performed with bilateral dedicated internal and external carotid injections. Dural AV fistulas are classically fed via external carotid branches. Pial arterial supply to dAVFs is very rare and should cause the diagnosis to be questioned.

PATHOLOGY AND CLINICAL CORRELATION Dural AV fistulas usually present in middle to older age patients. Adult-type dAVFs are caused by partial or complete revascularization of a previously thrombosed dural venous sinus. Clinically, the vast majority of dAVFs are simple fistulas and follow a benign course. Aggressive lesions are commonly associated with retrograde leptomeningeal venous drainage (RLVD) which is a response to high flow and venous congestion. This condition can be demonstrated on MRI and angiography by a PPP as in the companion case above. Ninety-eight percent of dAVFs without RLVD have a benign course. Location is also considered when evaluating the nature of a dAVF, with tentorial lesions commonly showing aggressive features.

Benign dAVF presentation often relates to location and includes tinnitus, cranial nerve palsies, and/or signs related to venous congestion in the orbit. Intracranial dAVFs associated with RLVD may have similar presentation or may present with intracranial haemorrhage, focal neurological defect, seizure, encephalopathic syndromes, dementia, or Parkinsonism.

Treatment often consists of observation with benign dAVFs. Aggressive lesions can be treated by endovascular obstruction, surgical resection, and/or with stereotactic radiation therapy.

TEACHING PEARLS
➤ *Objective pulsatile tinnitus can be caused by a multitude of factors, many of which can be diagnosed by the combination of MRI and MRA.*
➤ *When evaluating dAVFs, it is important to consider location and the presence of RLVD in assessing the benign or aggressive nature of the lesion.*
➤ *Adult type dAVFs are the result of revascularization of a previously thrombosed venous sinus.*

REFERENCES
Davies MA, *et al.* (1997). The natural history and management of intracranial dural arteriovenous fistulas, 1: benign lesion. *Intervent Neuroradiol* 3:295–302.
Davies MA, *et al.* (1997). The natural history and management of intracranial dural arteriovenous fistulas, 2: aggressive lesion. *Intervent Neuroradiol* 3:303–11.
Shin EJ, Lalwani AK, Dowd CF (2000). Role of angiography in the evaluation of patients with pulsatile tinnitus. *Laryngoscope* 110(11):1916–20.
Willinsky R, *et al.* (1999). Tortuous, enlarged pial veins in intracranial dural arteriovenous fistulas: correlation with presentation, location, and MR findings in 122 patients. *AJNR* 20:1031–6.

12 A patient presents with syncope, and the following images are obtained (**12A, B**).
i. What vessel is absent in image **12A**?
ii. What is the difference in MRA technique between the two images above?
iii. What is the treatment for subclavian steal?

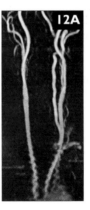 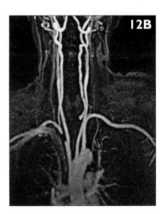

12 DIAGNOSIS Subclavian steal syndrome.

IMAGING FINDINGS The two dimensional time-of-flight (2D TOF) MRA image (**12A**) demonstrates normal carotid arteries bilaterally. The right vertebral artery is not identified on this sequence (**i**). The left vertebral artery appears normal. Contrast enhanced MRA (**12B**) of the same patient acquired at the same time as the 2D TOF sequence shows all four vessels with normal caliber (**ii**). However, there is a focal stenosis involving the proximal aspect of the right subclavian artery between its origin and the origin of the right vertebral artery.

DIFFERENTIAL DIAGNOSIS The initial determination to make is whether of not the lack of visualization of the right vertebral artery on the 2-D TOF sequence is due to technical causes. If it is truly absent, the differential includes congenital hypoplasia or occlusion (including postdissection thrombosis). Finally, reversed (craniocaudal) flow is also nonvisualized on 2D TOF sequences, and this diagnosis is consistent with the findings on the contrast enhanced MRA.

The explanation for the findings requires a basic understanding of TOF technique. In 2D TOF, a travelling saturation band is placed superior to the image plane and serves to obliterate all signal produced by flow that traverses the saturation band before the imaged plane, thus 'filtering out' all flow in the craniocaudal direction (usually venous). This process is repeated sequentially through the neck and produces a composite image of flow in the infero-superior direction only. Thus, in this case, the right vertebral artery is patent but there is retrograde flow in the vessel producing a subclavian steal.

PATHOLOGY AND CLINICAL CORRELATION Subclavian steal syndrome is a pathophysiologic process by which blood is preferentially diverted away from the brain retrogradely down the vertebral artery (usually the left) and into the subclavian artery, due to lower resistance along this pathway as opposed to the cerebral capillary bed. The lower resistance in the arm is commonly due to a focal high-grade stenosis of the proximal subclavian artery causing decreased distal pressure.

Subclavian steal is most commonly asymptomatic (greater than 90% of the time in several studies) or presents with symptoms of arm claudication secondary to the precipitating subclavian stenosis. However, patients occasionally present with symptoms related to vertebrobasilar insufficiency such as vertigo, ataxia, or visual disturbances. These findings can be exacerbated by arm activity.

When indicated by unequivocal posterior circulation or arm ischaemia, several treatment options exist. Surgical vascular transposition, bypass of the subclavian stenosis, or percutaneous transluminal angioplasty (with or without stent placement) are the most common therapies (**iii**). After the proximal subclavian stenosis is addressed, pressure increases appropriately within the more distal subclavian at the vertebral artery origin. Vascular resistance is then greater than that of the cerebral capillary bed and vertebral artery flow reverts to the normal antegrade direction.

TEACHING PEARLS
➤ *Retrograde flow in the vertebral artery is the radiographic hallmark of subclavian steal.*
➤ *Most subclavian steal cases are asymptomatic.*
➤ *Therapy involves treatment of the proximal subclavian stenosis.*

REFERENCES
Taylor CL, Selman WR, Ratcheson RA (2002). Steal affecting the central nervous system. *Neurosurgery* **50**(4):679–89.
van Grimberge F, *et al.* (2000). Role of magnetic resonance in the diagnosis of subclavian steal syndrome. *J Magn Reson Imaging* **12**:339–42.

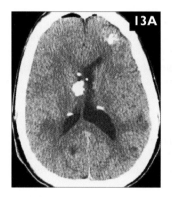 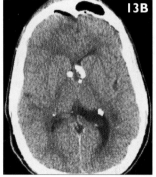

13 A 19-year-old male presents, recently status post surgery (**13A, B**). The patient has a long history of seizures.
i. What do the hyperdensities represent and where are they located?
ii. What is the diagnosis?

13 **DIAGNOSIS** Tuberous sclerosis complex (TSC).

IMAGING FINDINGS Images **13A, B** demonstrate multiple calcified subependymal nodules in the body and atrium of the lateral ventricle bilaterally. The larger masses at the right (**13A**) and left (**13B**) foramen of Monro represent subependymal giant cell astrocytomas and the lesion in the left frontal lobe represents a subcortical tuber (i). Findings are consistent with TSC (ii). Note the small amount of pneumocephalus adjacent to the frontal lobes related to recent craniotomy.

DIFFERENTIAL DIAGNOSIS Differential diagnosis of calcified periventricular lesions includes tuberous sclerosis, neurocysticercosis, the TORCH infections (Question 51), and metastasis (including ovarian cancer). (See Question **51** for a full discussion.)

PATHOLOGY AND CLINICAL CORRELATION Tuberous sclerosis complex (Bourneville–Pringle syndrome) is an inherited condition characterized histologically by calcified subependymal nodules, subependymal giant cell astrocytomas, and cortical/subcortical tubers. The classic clinical triad is: (1) seizures ('fits'), (2) facial angiofibromas ('zits'), and mental retardation ('nitwits'). Surgery is contemplated if a particular tuber can be implicated in seizure activity, or if the subependmyal giant cell astrocytoma obstructs the foramen of Munro. Extracranial manifestations are common and include angiomyolipomas (AMLs) of the kidney, cardiac rhabdomyomas, and lymphangioleiomyomatosis of the lung. Routine surveillance is typically with unenhanced MRI scanning.

TEACHING PEARLS
➤ *TSC is an inherited disorder with hamartomas in multiple organs.*
➤ *Cerebral manifestations include calcified subependymal nodules, subependymal giant cell astrocytomas, cortical/subcortical tubers, and radial white matter lesions along lines of neuronal migration.*
➤ *It presents with a classical clinical triad: facial angiofibromas, mental retardation, and seizures.*

REFERENCES
Altman NR, Purser RK, Post MJ (1988). Tuberous sclerosis: characteristics at CT and MR imaging. *Radiology* 167:527–32.
Seidenwurm DJ, Barkovich AJ (1992). Understanding tuberous sclerosis. *Radiology* 183:23–4.

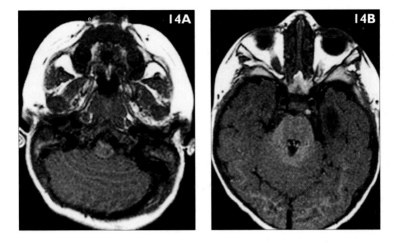

14 A child presents with developmental delay.
i. What type of MRI sequence is demonstrated (**14A, B**)?
ii. What structure is abnormal in the images above?

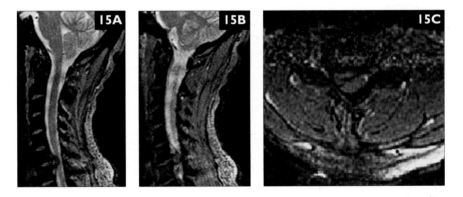

15 A 40-year-old male patient presents with pain and numbness in the middle finger of his right hand.
i. What does the sagittal T2 STIR image (**15A, B**) show?
ii. What effects are seen on the axial T2-weighted image (**15C**)?
iii. What nerve is likely compressed?

14 Diagnosis Rhomboencephalosynapsis.

Imaging findings Two axial T1-weighted images are presented for evaluation (notice bright subcutaneous fat and dark CSF) (i). The cerebellum is markedly abnormal (ii). There is fusion of the cerebellar hemispheres involving both grey and white matter. Transverse cerebellar diameter is reduced. Note the 'keyhole'-shaped 4th ventricle.

Differential diagnosis Findings reveal congenital fusion of the cerebellum. The only reasonable differential consideration would be congenital vermian hypoplasia.

Pathology and clinical correlation Rhomboencephalosynapsis is an extremely rare congenital fusion of the cerebellar hemispheres associated with decreased cerebellar transverse dimension and a 'keyhole'-shaped 4th ventricle. This is caused by an early induction failure of normal midline development. Findings are usually associated with supratentorial abnormalities. Children are usually picked up early in life after they are imaged due to ataxia, developmental delay, or seizures. Associated psychiatric disturbances have also been reported. Prognosis is affected by the number and type of additional abnormalities, but most children have a shortened lifespan.

Teaching pearls
➤ *Rhomboencephalosynapsis is an extremely rare congenital fusion of the cerebellum.*
➤ *Findings are often associated with other supratentorial abnormalities.*

References
Demaerel P, *et al.* (2004). Partial rhomboencephalosynapsis. *AJNR* **25**(1):29–31.
Toelle SP, *et al.* (2002). Rhomboencephalosynapsis: clinical findings and neuroimaging in 9 children. *Neuropediatrics* **33**:209–14.
Utsonomiya H, *et al.* (1998). Rhomboencephalosynapsis: cerebellar embryogenesis. *AJNR* **19**(3):547–9.

15 Diagnosis Right C6/7 disc herniation.

Imaging findings A large subligamentous disc herniation compresses the right side of the cord at C6/7 (i) and narrows the right neural foramen (ii). The C7 nerve is likely compressed (iii).

Pathology and clinical correlation A disc herniation is characterized by a focal protuberance of the disc margin. In the cervical spine, this is most common at C5/6 or C6/7 levels. Herniated disc fragments may remain subligamentous or may penetrate the posterior longitudinal ligament. They may migrate superior or inferior to the disc space. Long-standing disc herniations may calcify. Close assessment for cord compression or neural foramina stenosis is required.

TEACHING PEARL

➤ *The C6 nerve root is compressed by a C5/6 disc herniation and the C7 nerve root by a C6/7 disc herniation.*

REFERENCE

Abbed KM, Coumans JV (2007). Cervical radiculopathy: pathophysiology, presentation, and clinical evaluation. *Neurosurgery* 60(1 Suppl 1):S28–34.

---

16 A 34-year-old female presents with back pain and leg weakness, and the following image is obtained (**16A**).
i. What is the finding on this sagittal T2-weighted image of the spine?
ii. Is it abnormal?

DIFFERENTIAL DIAGNOSIS
Images **16B–D**.

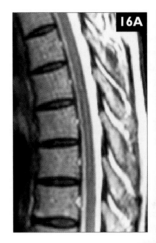
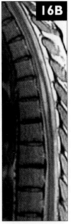
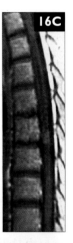
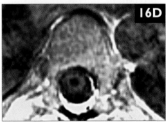

16 DIAGNOSIS Gibb's artifact.

IMAGING FINDINGS Image **16A** demonstrates a thin line of T2 hyperintensity extending longitudinally within the spinal cord (**i**).

DIFFERENTIAL DIAGNOSIS The differential diagnosis (**ii**) for this finding includes:
- Gibb's artifact (**16A**).
- Syringohydromyelia (**16B–D**).

PATHOLOGY AND CLINICAL CORRELATION Although a detailed discussion of physics is beyond the scope of this text, the imaging pattern of alternating bright lines parallel and adjacent to an interface of abrupt signal change (such as at the interface of cerebrospinal fluid [CSF] and the spinal cord) represents a manifestation of Gibb's artifact, also known as truncation artifact. The imaging appearance is related to the Fourier Transform, an integral part of the MR raw data processing algorithm, which has trouble resolving a sharp change in signal intensity without introducing alternating spikes on each side of the sharp transition, which we see as the bands of alternating signal intensity. Because it is inherent to the algorithm, Gibb's phenomenon is always present, but careful selection of imaging parameters can help to minimize the effect.

Images **16B–D** (sagittal T2, sagittal T1, axial T1, respectively) demonstrate an example of syringohydromyelia of the cervical cord, with a T1 hypointense/T2 hyperintense cleft within the spinal cord. Axial images help to demonstrate the precise location within the cord.

TEACHING PEARLS
- *Gibb's or truncation artifact can mimic pathology; look carefully for a characteristic pattern of alternating bright and dark signal lines that are adjacent to and parallel to an interface.*
- *Syringohydromyelia is a basket term for a cystic cord cavity that encompasses both hydromyelia (dilatation of the central canal of the spinal cord) and syringomyelia (which is separate from the central canal); because it is difficult to separate these entities with imaging alone, the term syringohydromyelia is used.*
- *Aetiologies of syringohydromyelia include trauma, Chiari I/II malformation, basilar invagination, or idiopathic.*
- *If one suspects syringohydromyelia, it is important to obtain contrast-enhanced images to exclude the possibility of spinal cord neoplasm, including the entire length of the abnormality.*

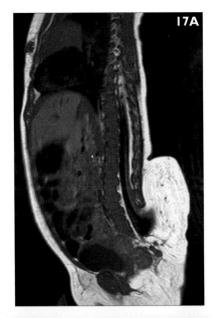

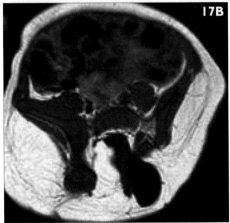

17 A neonate presents with a soft, nontender mass above the intergluteal crease. An MRI was performed (**17A, B**).

i. What abnormal tissue is demonstrated within the spinal canal?

ii. How did it get there?

iii. What is the most common differential diagnosis and how can it be distinguished?

17 **DIAGNOSIS** Lipomyelomeningocoele.

IMAGING FINDINGS The sacral subcutaneous fat is more prominent than usual, comprising a diffuse lipoma, which extends through a spina bifida dysraphic defect into the right side of the spinal canal (i). Here it is adherent to the right side of the neural placode. The lipoma-placode interface extends into a posterior meningocoele.

DIFFERENTIAL DIAGNOSIS
- Lipomyelocoele.
- Terminal myelocystocoele.
- Meningocoele.
- Sacrococcygeal teratoma.
- Caudal agenesis with overgrowth of fatty tissue.

PATHOLOGY AND CLINICAL CORRELATION Lipomyelomeningocoeles arise as an abnormality of primary neurulation (ii). The cutaneous ectoderm separates prematurely from the neuroectoderm, allowing access of mesenchyme into the canal. This differentiates into fatty tissue. By contrast, with a lipomyelocoele, the placode-lipoma interface lies inside the spinal canal, without prominent expansion of the subarachnoid spaces (iii).

Lipomyelomeningocoeles present at birth as a skin-covered lumbosacral mass. Nontreated infants develop lower limb and urinary symptoms.

TEACHING PEARLS
➢ *Spinal dysraphisms may be associated with a subcutaneous mass, commonly a lipoma.*
➢ *The lipomyelocoele and lipomyelomeningocoele can be differentiated from each other by the location of the placode-lipoma interface.*

REFERENCE
Rossi A, *et al.* (2004). Imaging in spine and spinal cord malformations. *Eur J Radiol* 50 (2):177–200.

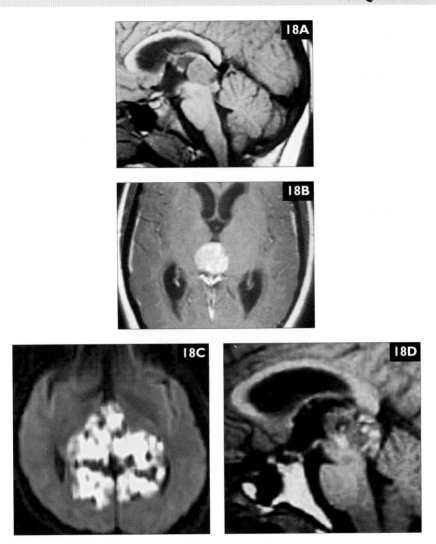

18 A 7-year-old girl presents with vomiting, and the following images are obtained (18A, B).
i. Where is this lesion located?
ii. How would you describe the enhancement pattern?
iii. What is the differential diagnosis for a mass in this area of the brain?

DIFFERENTIAL DIAGNOSIS Images 18C, D.

18 **DIAGNOSIS** Pineoblastoma.

IMAGING FINDINGS Images **18A, B** (sagittal T1, axial contrast-enhanced T1, respectively) demonstrate a T1 hypointense, homogeneously enhancing mass of the pineal gland (**i,ii**). There is compression of the aqueduct causing hydrocephalus with enlarged occipital and frontal horns.

DIFFERENTIAL DIAGNOSIS The differential diagnosis of a pineal region mass includes:
- Pineoblastoma (**18A, B**).
- Pineocytoma.
- Germinoma (see Question 38).
- Teratoma (**18D**, sagittal T1).
- Embryonal cell carcinoma.
- Choriocarcinoma.
- Metastases.
- Meningioma.
- Epidermoid (**18C**, axial DWI).
- Pineal cyst.

The high signal in DWI in **18C** is diagnostic for epidermoid cyst. The teratoma in **18D** is a heterogenous complex mass containing hypointense cystic and hyperintense fatty foci.

PATHOLOGY AND CLINICAL CORRELATION Pineoblastoma is a highly malignant WHO grade 4 primitive embryonal tumour of the pineal gland. About 30 % of patients present with spinal dissemination, which makes the prognosis of pineoblastoma dismal, with a median survival of about 20 months. Treatment is surgical resection with cranio-spinal radiation and chemotherapy. Detection of a pineal region mass mandates complete screening of the spine for drop metastasis.

TEACHING PEARLS
➤ *Pineal mass in men: 80% is germinoma.*
➤ *Pineal mass in women: 50% is pineal cell tumour (pineocytoma or pineoblastoma), 50% germinoma (See Question 38).*
➤ *Heterogenous pineal mass is often associated with necrosis, haemorrhage, and peripherally displaced calcification.*
➤ *Poor prognosis is due to cerebrospinal fluid dissemination.*
➤ *Symptoms include increased intracranial pressure and/or Parinaud syndrome (paralysis of upward gaze).*
➤ *Median patient age is 3 years.*

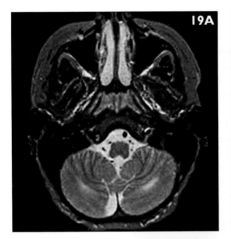
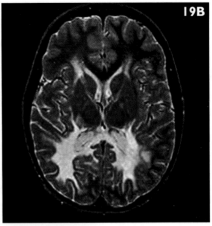
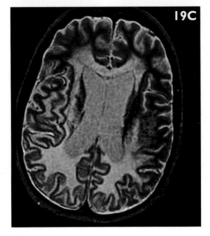

19 A 10-year-old boy presents with Addison's disease, behaviour problems, and decreasing mental function. An MRI of the brain was performed (**19A, B**).
i. What are the findings?
ii. What does the follow-up MR show 6 months later (**19C**)?
iii. What is the likely diagnosis?

19 DIAGNOSIS Adrenoleukodystrophy (ALD) (iii).

IMAGING FINDINGS The T2-weighted axial MR reveals the classic imaging findings of confluent symmetric hyperintensity within parietal–occipital white matter extending across the splenium of corpus callosum. This case also shows less severe changes surrounding the frontal horns, with patchy signal hyperintensity within the limbs of the internal capsules. The cerebellar white matter also shows T2 hyperintense white matter changes (i).

Follow-up imaging was performed 6 months later, by which time the patient had undergone a marked symptomatic decline, with development of seizures and spastic quadriplegia. T2-weighted axial MR shows marked progression in white matter disease with more extensive changes seen within central and subcortical white matter, now also involving the genu of corpus callosum. Diffuse progressive atrophy is present (ii).

Predominately posterior white matter involvement occurs in 80% of patients. CT hypodensity, MR T1 hypointensity and T2 hyperintensity are seen in affected areas, reflecting underlying demyelination. Contrast administration reveals enhancement of the lateral margins of the T2 signal changes, corresponding to an area of active demyelination.

DIFFERENTIAL DIAGNOSIS The broad differential diagnosis for white matter changes includes multiple sclerosis, ischaemia, and toxic and metabolic aetiologies. The rapid progression and pattern of change over 6 months is supportive of the latter. In this particular case, which shows the classic pattern of ALD, the differential diagnosis is limited. Another perioxisomal disorder, acyl CoA oxidase defiency, can show a similar pattern, but presents earlier in both sexes.

PATHOLOGY AND CLINICAL CORRELATION ALD is an X-linked recessive perioxisomal disorder, resulting from a mutation in the ALD gene. This causes impaired transport of very long chain fatty acids, and impaired myelin structure. The commonest clinical form of ALD is the childhood cerebral form, where boys present between the ages of 5 and 12 with behaviour problems, reducing mental function, and visual and hearing problems, which later progresses to motor symptoms and ataxia. Some may show features of Addison disease. Histologically, the brain shows symmetric inflammatory demyelination, most severe in the posterior white matter, which extends across the splenium of the corpus callosum. Cerebellar and optic nerve involvement is common.

TEACHING PEARLS
- *ALD presents most commonly in male children.*
- *White matter changes are more predominately posteriorly, extend across the splenium of corpus callosum, and may show peripheral enhancement.*
- *White matter changes are progressive.*

REFERENCE
Barkovich AJ (2005). *Pediatric Neuroimaging*, 4th edn. Lippincott, Williams and Wilkins, Philadelphia.

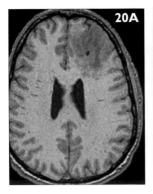
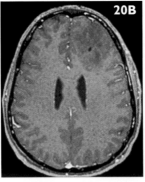
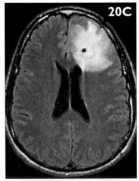

20 A 46-year-old female with headaches for several weeks, presents with seizures and the following images are obtained (20A–C).

i. Where is the lesion located and which structure is spared?

ii. What are the signal characteristics, morphology, and enhancement pattern?

iii. What could the hypointense 'dot' within the lesion represent?

iv. What is the differential diagnosis for a lesion in this location?

DIFFERENTIAL DIAGNOSIS
Images 20D–G.

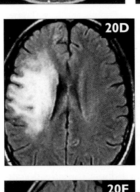
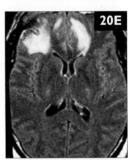
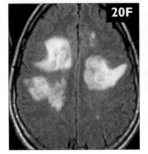
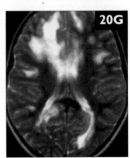

20 DIAGNOSIS Oligodendroglioma.

IMAGING FINDINGS Images 20A–C (sagittal T1, axial post-contrast T1, axial FLAIR, respectively) demonstrate a T1 hypointense, FLAIR hyperintense, essentially nonenhancing lesion located in the subcortical and deep white matter (WM) of the left frontal lobe, sparing the grey matter (**i, ii**). A well-demarcated round focus of low signal on all pulse sequences, best seen on the FLAIR sequence, could represent a fluid-filled cyst (one should correlate with T2 to determine fluid content), susceptibility artifact from metal, old haemorrhage, or calcification, or a flow void (**iii**).

DIFFERENTIAL DIAGNOSIS The differential diagnosis (**iv**) of a subcortical WM lesion in an immunocompetent patient includes:

- Low-grade astrocytoma.
- Oligodendroglioma (**20A–C**).
- Glioblastoma multiforme.
- Anaplastic astrocytoma.
- Gliomatosis cerebri (see Question **26**).
- Demyelination.
- Tumefactive multiple sclerosis (MS) (**20**, axial FLAIR).
- Tumefactive acute disseminated encephalomyelitis (ADEM) (**20G**, axial FLAIR).
- Progressive multifocal leukoencephalopathy (PML) (**20D**, axial FLAIR).
- Neurosarcoid (**20E**, axial FLAIR).
- Cerebritis.
- Plus: see differential diagnosis of peripherally located supratentorial mass without mass effect (Question **5**).

Focal lesions centred in WM have a broad differential diagnosis, and distinguishing among the many possibilities requires consideration of the clinical history and the imaging characteristics, including the presence of enhancement and mass effect. When confronted with multiple periventricular, deep WM, and subcortical WM lesions without enhancement (a very common finding), the differential possibilities include small vessel ischaemic change (the most likely diagnosis), demyelination, Lyme disease, vasculitis, and sequela of previous migraine. In this case, we have a single dominant lesion, which refocuses the differential: the two largest categories to consider are neoplasm and demyelination, which are presented above in the first two groups. Tumefactive MS and ADEM (**20F, G**) have relatively little mass effect for the amount of signal abnormality present, and MR may demonstrate additional WM lesions separate from the mass.

PML presents as a nonenhancing, often bilateral WM lesion, less commonly unilateral as in **20D** (see Question **21**). Neurosarcoid (**20E**) is often located in the basal cisterns involving optic chiasm, hypothalamus, infundibulum, and cranial nerves. Neurosarcoid is typically a multifocal and dural-based mass in contrast to oligodendroglioma.

PATHOLOGY AND CLINICAL CORRELATION Oligodendrogliomas are slowly growing but infiltrating cortical/subcortical tumours. They are the tumour type most likely to calcify (nodular or clumped calcification in 70–90%), although their relative rarity makes a particular calcified lesion more likely to represent a glioma. Cystic degeneration is common and enhancement is variable. The majority are supratentorial (85%). They are often located in the frontal lobe. A portion of oligodendrogliomas are anaplastic, although the distinction may require biopsy as imaging features are not diagnostic. Patients are typically between 40 and 50 years old and have relatively long-standing history of headaches and seizures. With surgical resection, radiation, and chemotherapy, the median survival rate is 10 years. Prognosis is typically better than that associated with astrocytomas of the same grade.

TEACHING PEARLS
- ➤ *A frontal lobe calcified mass in a middle-aged adult is a typical presentation of oligodendroglioma. Look also for cortical expansion, which favours oligodendroglioma.*
- ➤ *Differentiation between low-grade (WHO grade 2) and anaplastic oligodendroglioma (WHO grade 3) is not reliable with imaging alone.*
- ➤ *There is better correlation between tumour grade and cerebral blood volume (CBV) than between tumour grade and enhancement, although even low-grade oligodendrogliomas can have false-positive high CBV.*
- ➤ *New enhancement in previously nonenhancing oligodendroglioma often indicates malignant progression.*

REFERENCES
Koeller KK, Rushing EJ (2005). Oligodendroglioma and its variants: radiologic–pathologic correlation. *Radiographics* 25:1669–88.
Osborn AG, *et al.* (2004). *Brain*. Amirsys, Salt Lake City, Chapter I, pp. 6, 52–5, 92–5.

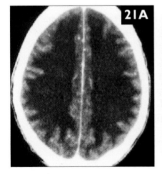 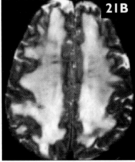 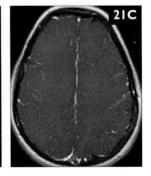

21 The following images are obtained from a patient with HIV (**21A–C**).
i. Where is the lesion located? Which compartments are involved?
ii. Which sequences are shown and what are the signal characteristics of the lesion?
iii. What is the major differential consideration?

21 DIAGNOSIS   Progressive multifocal leukoencephalopathy (PML).

IMAGING FINDINGS   Image 21A–C (unenhanced CT, axial T2, and axial contrast-enhanced T1, respectively) show a confluent lesion infiltrating the entire centrum semiovale and the subcortical U-fibres bilaterally, without causing mass effect (**i**). The area is nonenhancing and T2 hyperintense. The typical pattern of PML, as in this case, is nonenhancing, multifocal, unilateral or bilateral asymmetric areas of T2 hyperintensity without enhancement (**ii**).

DIFFERENTIAL DIAGNOSIS   The major differential considerations in an HIV patient even before imaging include infection or lymphoma; distinguishing these entities is important for guiding therapy, although a common algorithm is to treat for infection and re-image to gauge treatment response. The lesions in this differential involve the white matter (WM) and are unlikely to be confused with TB or lymphoma based on imaging, but they are important to consider when reviewing images from an HIV-positive patient.
- PML.
- HIV encephalitis.
- Cytomegalovirus (CMV) encephalitis.

TEACHING PEARLS
➤ *PML presents on imaging with patchy, nonenhancing often confluent and bilateral WM lesion with involvement of the subcortical U-fibres, most often posterior.*
➤ *In a patient with HIV and subcortical WM abnormality, favour PML over other HIV-related diseases.*
➤ *Major differential considerations include HIV encephalopathy (usually symmetric and associated with atrophy), or CMV encephalitis (often shows subependymal enhancement) (**iii**).*
➤ *About 5% of AIDS patients acquire PML, caused by JC virus.*
➤ *PML is usually a fatal infection, with death occurring 6 months to 1 year after onset.*

REFERENCES
Graham CB, *et al.* (2000). Screening CT of the brain determined by CD4 count in HIV-positive patients presenting with headache. *Am J Neuroradiol* **21**:451–4.
Grossman RI, *et al.* (2003). *Neuroradiology*. Mosby, Philadelphia, pp. 347–8.

22 A 70-year-old male patient presents to accident and emergency with recent onset of right hemiparesis. A CT scan of his head was performed to rule out intracranial haemorrhage (22A).

i. What does the CT scan of the brain show?

ii. What is the other study (22B), how was it performed, and what does it show?

iii. What MR sequences may be helpful in further evaluating the patient?

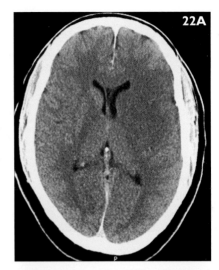

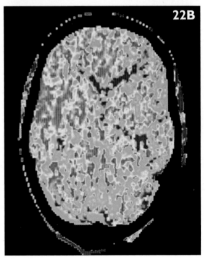

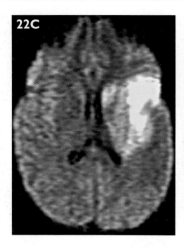
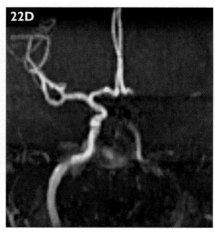

22 **Diagnosis** Acute left middle cerebral artery infarction

Imaging findings There is decreased attenuation of the left basal ganglia (**22A**), with a loss of the normal contrast between the lentiform nucleus and the internal capsule. This change extends peripherally towards the left insula. The left caudate head also shows low attenuation (**i**).

The colour map of mean transit time (**22B**), shows the findings from a CT perfusion study (**ii**). This technique can be very helpful in evaluating the acute stroke patient by providing a measure of brain perfusion. Cerebral blood flow, cerebral blood volume, and mean transit time of blood flow to brain can all be derived and are commonly presented as colour maps, to allow comparison between different regions of the brain. The colour map in this patient shows a prolonged mean transit time in the left basal ganglia (the colour scale shows a short mean transit time as red and a prolonged time as blue). This suggests that cerebral perfusion is reduced to this region of brain.

A diffusion-weighted MR sequence (**22C**) was performed, which revealed signal hyperintensity from diffusion restriction in the area of suspected ischaemia, in keeping with acute cerebral infarction (**iii**). An MR angiogram (**22D**) showed no flow within the left internal carotid artery, a result of occlusion. No flow was seen in the left middle cerebral artery, but the left anterior cerebral artery filled from the right anterior circulation.

Teaching pearls
➤ *Perfusion studies allow detection of early cerebral ischaemia.*
➤ *Can be used with diffusion-weighted imaging to estimate the ischaemic penumbra.*

Reference
Shetty SK, Lev MH (2005). CT perfusion in acute stroke. *Neuroimaging Clin N Am* **15**(3):481–501; ix Review.

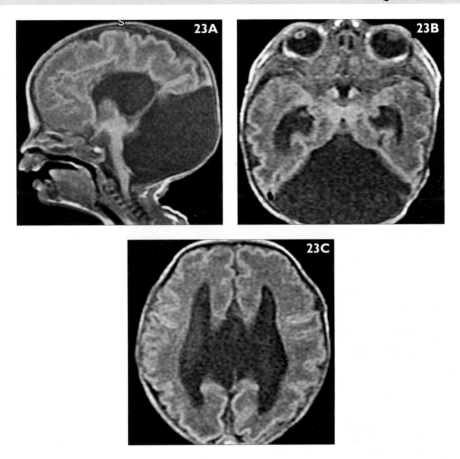

23 An infant presents in the first few months of life with seizures and developmental delay. An MRI of the brain was performed, and the following images obtained (23A–C).
i. What is the primary abnormality?
ii. Are there any associated anomalies?

23 **DIAGNOSIS** Dandy–Walker malformation (i).

IMAGING FINDINGS The sagittal (**23A**) and axial T1-weighted images (**23B, C**) show the classic findings of a Dandy–Walker malformation. The posterior fossa is markedly enlarged and filled with a large cerebrospinal fluid (CSF) cyst that communicates with the 4th ventricle. The tentorium is elevated. The cerebellar vermis is hypogenetic and hypoplastic cerebellar hemispheres are pushed laterally by the cyst. The brainstem is compressed anteriorly. There is evidence of hydrocephalus, a finding in around 90% of affected patients by the time of diagnosis, and also corpus callosal agenesis (found in around 30% of patients with Dandy–Walker syndrome). Salient imaging features of the latter on axial imaging include parallel lateral ventricles and a high riding 3rd ventricle, which extends between the lateral ventricles (**ii**).

PATHOLOGY AND CLINICAL CORRELATION Developmental cerebellar abnormalities can be classified as either hypoplastic (small but otherwise normal appearing) or dysplastic (abnormal appearing). The Dandy–Walker malformation is the severe end of a spectrum of hypoplasia of the cerebellar vermis.

TEACHING PEARL
➤ *Dandy–Walker malformation is commonly associated with other intracranial developmental anomalies.*

REFERENCE
Patel S, Barkovich AJ (2002). Analysis and classification of cerebellar malformations. *AJNR* **23**(7):1074–87.

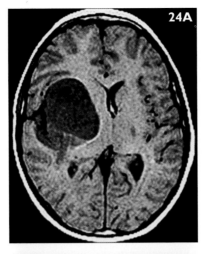

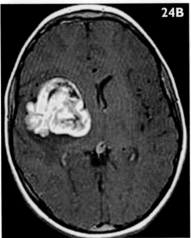

24 An 11-year-old child presents with seizures. The following images are obtained (**24A, B**).

i. Are most childhood tumours supra- or infratentorial?

ii. What is the most common cerebral tumour of childhood?

iii. What is a common mechanism of spread for paediatric cerebral neoplasms?

24 DIAGNOSIS Supratentorial primitive neuroectodermal tumour (S-PNET).

IMAGING FINDINGS This case demonstrates a well-defined large mass centred within the right cerebral hemisphere adjacent to the sylvian fissure. The mass shows hypointensity on T1 imaging and heterogeneous enhancement with relatively little surrounding oedema.

In general, S-PNETs show marked variability in imaging characteristics. The lesions are usually well-circumscribed and are found within the supratentorial cortex, thalamus, pineal region, and suprasellar cistern. This is in sharp distinction to most childhood tumours which are found in the posterior fossa (i). Tumours are usually large at presentation. Enhancement is heterogeneous and calcification is common. Masses can be either completely solid or have cystic components. There is often intratumoural restricted diffusion.

DIFFERENTIAL DIAGNOSIS Imaging findings are nonspecific. The differential diagnosis in young children typically includes supratentorial epenymoma, S-PNET, oligodendroglioma, and atypical teratoid/rhabdoid tumour. Definitive diagnosis is achieved only following biopsy.

PATHOLOGY AND CLINICAL CORRELATION S-PNET and medulloblastoma (PNET-MB) are closely related, though distinct, tumours. Both show primitive embryonal cell origin. While medulloblastomas are the most common paediatric cerebral neoplasm (ii), S-PNETs are quite rare and represent <1% of all paediatric brain tumours. They are most commonly found in young children (mean age 5 years). S-PNETs are similar to medulloblastoma in their propensity for CSF dissemination (iii). Therefore, it is important to image the entire neuroaxis to evaluate for tumour spread. Treatment is by complete surgical resection as well as chemo- and radiation therapy. Prognosis is poor and significantly worse than medulloblastoma. Patients show a 5-year survival of 37% compared to 80–85% with medulloblastoma.

TEACHING PEARLS
➤ *S-PNET is a rare neoplasm of young children that is generally well-circumscribed in the supratentorial brain but is otherwise heterogeneous in imaging characteristics.*
➤ *Prognosis is dismal and significantly worse than the closely-related medulloblastoma.*

REFERENCES
Reddy AT (2001). Advances in biology and treatment of childhood brain tumours. *Curr Neurol Neurosci Rep* **1**(2):137–43.
Young-Poussaint T (2001). Magnetic resonance imaging of pediatric brain tumours: state of the art. *Topics in Magnetic Resonance Imaging* **12**(6):411–34.

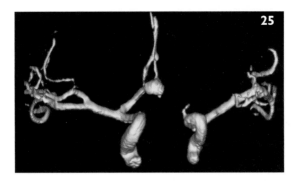

25 A 30-year-old female patient presents with a family history of cerebral aneurysm.
i. What type of examination is this (25)?
ii. What does it show?

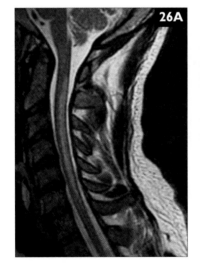

26 A 50-year-old woman presents with weakness and paresthesia of the lower limbs and the following images are obtained (26A–C).
i. What dietary deficiency may this patient have?
ii. Are the findings reversible?

25 DIAGNOSIS Anterior communicating aneurysm (ii).

IMAGING FINDINGS This 3T MR angiogram (volume rendered, MRA) (i) reveals a solitary berry aneurysm arising from the anterior communicating artery (ii).

PATHOLOGY AND CLINICAL CORRELATION The prevalence of intracranial aneurysm is estimated around 1% and 6% in adult postmortem series. Although most occur sporadically, there is an increased familial incidence of berry aneurysm. The most common site, is the anterior communicating/ anterior cerebral artery.

MRA is commonly performed either as a noninvasive (time-of-flight) or minimally invasive (contrast enhanced) study. It is an extremely useful diagnostic tool, often alleviating the need for conventional angiography, with its inherent risks including stroke. While computed tomography angiography (CTA) is currently more commonly used as a tool for diagnosing the acutely ruptured aneurysm (due largely to the important role of CT in diagnosing subarachnoid haemorrhage), MRA has an important role in screening for aneurysms, particularly in asymptomatic subjects.

TEACHING PEARL
➤ *CT and MR angiography are useful diagnostic techniques for the detection of cerebral aneurysms.*

REFERENCE
Wardlaw JM, White PM (2000). The detection and management of unruptured intracranial aneurysms. *Brain* **123**(2):205–21.

26 DIAGNOSIS Subacute combined degeneration of the cord secondary to vitamin B12 deficiency (i).

IMAGING FINDINGS Sagittal T2 FSE reveals a continuous long segment of T2 hyperintensity within the cervical cord, together with mild cord expansion. Axial T2 gradient echo images confirm that this is located within the posterior columns. Minimal enhancement of the cord is seen. Brain imaging may be normal or show nonspecific focal T2 hyperintensities. Imaging findings can resolve after B12 treatment (ii).

DIFFERENTIAL DIAGNOSIS This includes demyelination, ischaemia, and tumour.

PATHOLOGY AND CLINICAL CORRELATION Subacute combined degeneration of the cord occurs when chronic B12 deficiency causes demyelination and vacuolation of the myelin sheaths of the posterior columns of the spinal cord. This may progress to involve lateral and, less commonly, anterior columns. Gliosis and atrophy follows. Initial peripheral sensory symptoms may evolve to an ataxic paraplegia, if left untreated. The most common cause of vitamin B12 deficiency in the Western world is pernicious anaemia, an autoimmune gastritis resulting in a lack of instrinsic factor. Other causes include gastric surgery and malabsorption syndromes.

TEACHING PEARL
➤ *Prompt diagnosis of subacute combined degeneration of the cord is important as early treatment can reverse clinical (and radiological) findings.*

REFERENCE
Hemmer B, *et al.* (1998). Subacute combined degeneration: clinical, electrophysiological and magnetic resonance imaging findings. *J Neurol Neurosurg Psychiatry* 65:822–7.

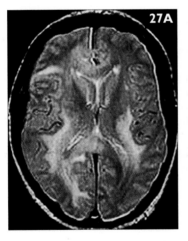 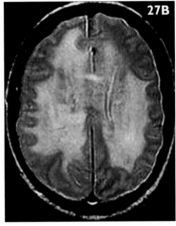

27 A patient presents with slowly progressing left-sided weakness and persistent headache. The following images are obtained (27A, B).
i. What is the predominant distribution of the abnormal signal?
ii. Identify an important finding in the midline that will help limit the differential diagnosis.
iii. Name several symmetric lesions affecting the brain.

27 **Diagnosis** Gliomatosis cerebri (GC).

Imaging findings There is diffuse signal abnormality infiltrating throughout the white matter of the cerebral hemispheres bilaterally (i). Abnormal signal is clearly seen crossing the corpus callosum both anterior and posteriorly (ii).

Differential diagnosis The most common symmetric white matter lesions of brain include chronic microvascular changes, encephalitis, demyelinating disease, vasculitis, and leukoencephalopathy (iii). GC should always be considered though it is significantly less common than the other etiologies in the differential. However, involvement of the corpus callosum should raise GC to the top of the list in this case.

Pathology and clinical correlation The World Health Organization defines GC as a diffusely infiltrative glioma. GC can be present with or without a dominant mass but must involve two or more lobes. Findings on MRI include diffuse T2 hyperintensity throughout the white matter that usually extends into deep grey nuclei as well. Findings are often bilateral and symmetric. Though enhancement is usually absent, its presence has been correlated with higher grade lesions. Enlargement of affected structures is generally present.

Typical presentation is enigmatic as neuronal numbers and architecture are only minimally affected. GC affects all age groups and can be of varying histological grade. Prognosis in generally poor. Treatment options include radiation and chemotherapy as well as occasional surgical decompression.

Teaching pearls
➤ *GC is a diffusely infiltrating glioma with or without a dominant mass affecting white matter and deep grey nuclei, often bilaterally.*
➤ *Presentation is enigmatic as the normal cerebral architecture is preserved.*
➤ *All age groups are affected and prognosis is extremely poor.*

References
del Carpio-O'Donovan R, *et al.* (1996). Gliomatosis cerebri. *Radiology* 198:831–5.
Vates GE, *et al.* (2003). Gliomatosis cerebri: a review of 22 cases. *Neurosurgery* 53(2):261–71.

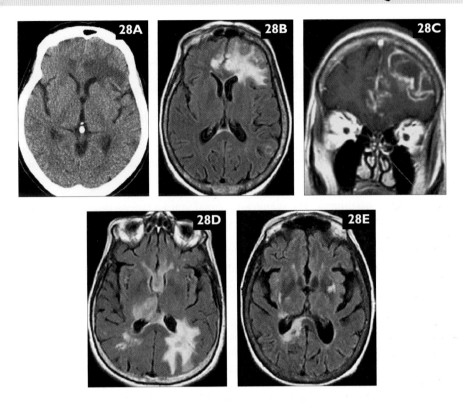

28 A 35-year-old male presents with seizures and history of AIDS, and the following images are obtained (**28A–C**).
i. Where is the lesion located?
ii. Which sequences are shown and what are the signal characteristics of the lesion?
iii. Even without imaging, what is the primary differential diagnosis and why is the distinction important?

DIFFERENTIAL DIAGNOSIS Images 28D, E.

28 DIAGNOSIS Tuberculosis (TB).

IMAGING FINDINGS Images 28A–C (axial unenhanced CT, axial FLAIR, coronal postcontrast T1, respectively) demonstrate a confluent well-defined lesion in the subcortical and deep white matter (WM) of the left frontal lobe (**i, ii**), causing mass effect with midline shift to the right. The lesion is hypodense on CT and shows peripheral rim enhancement around a hypointense (most likely necrotic) core after contrast administration on MR. Note also the leptomeningeal enhancement seen anteriorly along the midline, parenchymal signal abnormality, and enhancement in the medial aspect of the right frontal lobe, and a subtle area of FLAIR hyperintensity in the left temporal lobe.

DIFFERENTIAL DIAGNOSIS The major differential considerations in an HIV patient even before imaging include infection or lymphoma; distinguishing these entities is important for guiding therapy, although a common algorithm is to treat for infection and re-image to gauge treatment response (**iii**). The differential diagnosis of a leptomeningeal and parenchymal lesion in a immunocompromised patient includes:
• Tuberculosis.
• Lymphoma (**28D**, axial FLAIR).
• Toxoplasmosis.
• Abscess.
• Cryptococcosis (atypical) (**28E**, axial FLAIR).
Lymphoma (**28D**) shows strong enhancement and might be difficult to distinguish from TB. Involvement of the basal ganglia, periventricular WM, and ependymal surfaces would favour lymphoma. Toxoplasmosis would present as an enhancing lesion that would be expected to respond to anti-microbial therapy.

The typical appearance of an abscess is a rim-enhancing, T2 hyperintense structure with centrally restricted diffusion. Image **28E** shows multiple hyperintense lesions affecting the deep grey nuclei bilaterally, the splenium of the corpus callosum, and the WM surrounding the occipital horn of the right lateral ventricle. This represents cryptococcosis in a patient with AIDS. The most common fungal agent to involve the CNS in AIDS patients, *Cryptococcus* can present as a basilar meningitis, as large parenchymal lesions known as cryptococcomas, or as dilated perivascular spaces distended with organisms and mucoid material ('gelatinous pseudocysts').

PATHOLOGY AND CLINICAL CORRELATION TB is a granulomatous disease caused by *Mycobacterium tuberculosis* that shows CNS involvement in about 10% of cases. Intracranial TB presents either as a basilar meningitis and/or as localized CNS infection (tuberculoma). Tuberculoma can present in the following stages of evolution: noncaseating, caseating with solid centre, or caseating with necrotic centre. This case shows a caseating tuberculoma with peripheral rim enhancement and necrotic centre. Tuberculomas are typically multifocal, round- or oval-shaped masses, most commonly located in the parietal lobes. The incidence of TB has increased in recent years, particularly in conjunction with AIDS. About 15% of AIDS patients have CNS TB and in underdeveloped countries tuberculomas account for about 25% of all intracranial masses. Complications in CNS TB often include hydrocephalus, stroke, and seizures.

TEACHING PEARLS
➤ *The combination of basilar leptomeningeal disease and parenchymal lesions in an immunocompromised patient suggests TB.*
➤ *TB is re-emerging due to immigration from endemic areas and the increase of AIDS incidence.*
➤ *Be aware of complications such as hydrocephalus and stroke.*

REFERENCES
Graham CB, *et al.* (2000). Screening CT of the brain determined by CD4 count in HIV-positive patients presenting with headache. *Am J Neuroradiol* 21:451–4.
Grossman RI, *et al.* (2003). *Neuroradiology*. Mosby, Philadelphia, pp. 347–8.

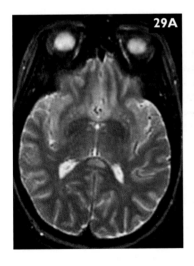

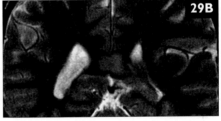

29 A 32-year-old female patient presents with a long-standing seizure disorder under good control with anti-epileptic medications. The following images are obtained (**29A, B**).
i. Where is the abnormal signal located?
ii. Name three entities known to cross midline cerebral structures.

29 DIAGNOSIS Anti-epileptic drug (AED)-related white matter changes.

IMAGING FINDINGS There is a well-defined elliptical focus of increased signal on T2-weighted axial and coronal images within the splenium of the corpus callosum (i).

DIFFERENTIAL DIAGNOSIS Very few cerebral lesions cross midline structures. The classical examples include glioblastoma multiforme, primary CNS lymphoma, and demyelinating disease (ii). Additional considerations may include trauma, infection, and metabolic abnormalities such as Machiafava–Bignami. In this case, the elliptical pattern of abnormal signal and the classic position of the abnormality centred within the splenium should raise concern for AED-related white matter disease.

PATHOLOGY AND CLINICAL CORRELATION Over the last 10 years there have been multiple reported cases of well marginated T2 hyperintensity centred within the splenium of the corpus callosum in seizure patients treated with AEDs. Initial reports focused on Dilantin (phenytoin); however, subsequent cases have been presented with patients treated with other anti-seizure medications. Though the aetiology of the signal abnormality is unknown, several hypotheses have been proposed. Current theories focus on direct toxicity from the offending medications or metabolic changes related to changes in drug levels or to the seizure activity itself.

Signal abnormality is confined to the splenium and shows mild expansion but no abnormal enhancement. There have been limited reports of transient diffusion restriction within such lesions. Cases have been noted to appear acutely and are noted to resolve completely in weeks to months. No symptoms have been directly correlated with the imaging abnormalities. Recognition is important in order to avoid unneeded additional testing.

TEACHING PEARL

➤ *Well-marginated elliptical T2 hyperintensity centred within the splenium of the corpus callosum in epileptic patients should raise suspicion for transient AED-related white matter changes.*

REFERENCES

Kim SS, *et al.* (1999). Focal lesion in the splenium of the corpus callosum in epileptic patients: anti-epileptic drug toxicity? *AJNR* **20**:125–9.

Oster J, *et al.* (2003). Brief communication: diffusion-weighted imaging abnormalities in the splenium after seizures. *Epilepsia* **44**:1–3.

Polster T, Hoppe M, Ebner A (2001). Transient lesion in the splenium of the corpus callosum: three further cases in epileptic patients and a pathalogical hypothesis. *J Neurol Neurosurg Psychiatry* **70**:459–63.

30 A 30-year-female patient presents with seizures. Surgical resection is contemplated.
i. What type of examination is shown (30)?
ii. What does it show?

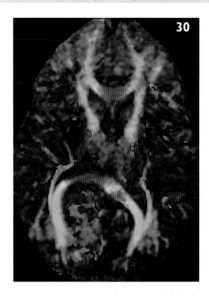

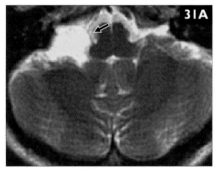

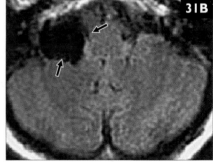

31 An abnormality was incidentally noted in a 45-year-old female on these T2-weighted (31A) and FLAIR (31B) images (arrows).
i. Where is the lesion located?
ii. What is the differential diagnosis? What sequence would help further narrow the differential?

30 DIAGNOSIS Low-grade glioma.

IMAGING FINDINGS Diffusion tensor imaging (DTI) (i) shows displacement of the splenium of the corpus callosum secondary to a mass (in this case a low-grade glioma) in the right occipital lobe (ii).

PATHOLOGY AND CLINICAL CORRELATION In some centres, DTI is used as a tool for planning tumour resection, often alongside functional MRI. Diffusion-weighted imaging allows detection of random water movement at a cellular level. With DTI, the directionality of this movement can be assessed, allowing detection of anisotropic white matter, which favours water diffusion along, rather than across, its myelin sheaths. Thus, the pathways of white matter tracts can be identified.

TEACHING PEARL
➤ *Early data suggest that DTI might be able to detect whether a tumour displaces or invades white matter tracts, important both surgically and prognostically.*

REFERENCE
Witwer BP, *et al.* (2002). Diffusion-tensor imaging of white matter tracts in patients with cerebral neoplasm. *J Neurosurg* **97**(3):568–75.

31 DIAGNOSIS Arachnoid cyst (AC).

IMAGING FINDINGS Images **31A, B** (T2 and FLAIR images) show a T2 hyperintense lesion in the right cerebellopontine angle (i) that matches CSF on the FLAIR image.

DIFFERENTIAL DIAGNOSIS The only important differential possibilities are AC versus epidermoid tumour. Diffusion-weighted imaging (DWI) would be useful to characterize this abnormality, as epidermoid tumours (solid) are associated with restricted diffusion (hyperintense DWI signal), and ACs (CSF) with elevated diffusion (hypointense DWI signal) (ii).

PATHOLOGY AND CLINICAL CORRELATION ACs are congenital and benign extra-axial cysts. These sharply-marginated extra-axial lesions will have imaging characteristics identical to CSF on CT and MR and will displace vessels and adjacent cortex. Lesions are most commonly found in the middle cranial fossa. They are most commonly asymptomatic and incidental, requiring no treatment, although associated symptoms are possible and dependent on location and size.

TEACHING PEARLS
➤ *CSF intensity on all MR sequences suggests AC.*
➤ *AC shows complete fluid attenuation on FLAIR sequence and no resticted diffusion on DWI sequences (ii).*
➤ *Location: 50% occur in the middle cranial fossa, 33% in the posterior fossa.*
➤ *Most patients do not require treatment.*

REFERENCES
Dutt SN, *et al.* (2002). Radiologic differentiation of intracranial epidermoids from arachnoid cysts. *Otol Neurotol* **23**:84–92.

Osborne AG, Preece MT (2006). Intracranial cysts: radiologic–pathologic correlation and imaging approach. *Radiology* **239**:650–64.

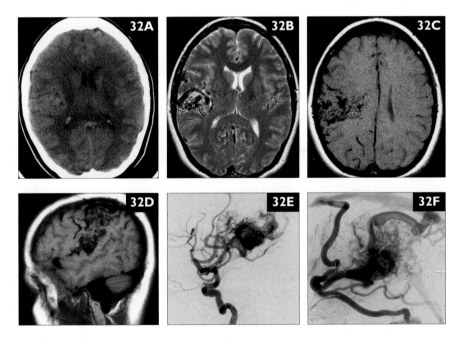

32 A patient presents with recent seizure and investigations are carried out (**32A–F**).
i. What do the dark regions within the right hemispheric mass represent on the MRI images (**32B–D**)?
ii. What is the central portion of this type of lesion called?
iii. Name several vascular malformations of the CNS.

32 **DIAGNOSIS** Arteriovenous malformation (AVM).

IMAGING FINDINGS There is faint hyperattenuation within the peripheral right frontal lobe on noncontrast head CT (**32A**). T2 (**32B**) and T1 (**32C, D**) MRI images demonstrate multiple serpentine dark vascular flow voids in the region (**i**). There is no suggestion of acute haemorrhage or mass effect. Arterial (**32E**) and capillary (**32F**) phases of a right common carotid conventional digital subtraction angiogram show a large tangle of vessels corresponding to the area of CT/MRI abnormality. Several early draining veins are seen extending superficially from the central vascular nidus (**ii**).

DIFFERENTIAL DIAGNOSIS Hyperattenuation on noncontrast head CT often represents haemorrhage or calcification. Other possibilities include hypercellular tumours or extremely vascular lesions (as in this case). Flow voids on MRI confirm a vascular malformation. There are multiple types of vascular malformations seen within the CNS. AVM, developmental venous anomaly (venous angioma), cavernous malformation, and capillary telangiectasia are the most common (**iii**). The feature that differentiates AVMs from these other, less ominous lesions is an absence of capillary development resulting in an abnormal connection of the corresponding artery and vein. This is demonstrated angiographically by a tangle of vessels (or nidus) draining into a large vein before the capillary phase has been seen. This finding confirms the diagnosis and essentially eliminates the other vascular malformations from the differential diagnosis.

PATHOLOGY AND CLINICAL CORRELATION Brain AVMs are characterized by an absence of capillary development. This may result in components of the AVM with direct arterial-to-venous connections known as fistulas, or with an intervening vascular bed made up of multiple abnormal small vessels (nidus). The incidence of AVMs is 0.14% of the general population which is significantly lower than that of intracranial sacular aneurysms. These congenital lesions usually present before age 40 years with haemorrhage (50%) or seizures (25%) as the most common presenting symptom. Haemorrhage is often related to intranidal aneurysm rupture and is estimated at approximately 2–4% per year, with the risk of recurrent haemorrhage being significantly higher for the first year following haemorrhage. The incidence of severe neurologic deficit or death is approximately 30–50% per haemorrhagic episode. In addition to haemorrhage, AVMs can lead to hypoperfusion of adjacent brain by shunting of blood through the relatively low resistance AVM rather than the adjacent, higher resistance, capillary beds.

AVMs are most commonly classified by the Spetzler–Martin grading system. Lesion size, location, and venous draining patterns are used to determine a grade of 1–5. These grades correspond to risk of surgical resection with lower grade lesions showing better outcomes. In addition to surgery, AVMs can be treated by focused radiotherapy and/or transcatheter embolization.

TEACHING PEARLS
> AVMs are characterized by the lack of development of normal capillaries.
> These lesions appear angiographically as a nidus of vessels with an early draining vein.
> The Spetzler–Martin grading system is used to estimate morbidity associated with surgical resection.
> Risk of haemorrhage is approximately 2–4% per year in untreated cases.

REFERENCES
Brown RD Jr, et al. (1988). The natural history of unruptured intracranial arteriovenous malformation. *J Neurosurg* **68**:352–7.
Spetzler RF, Martin NA (1986). A proposed grading system for arteriovenous malformations. *J Neurosurg* **65**:476–83.
Wallace RC, Bourekas EC (1998). Brain arteriovenous malformations. *Neuroimaging Clin N Am* 8(2):383–99.

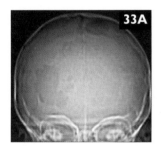

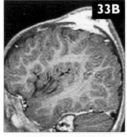

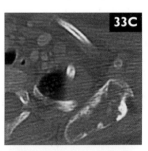

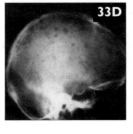

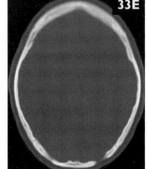

33 A 2-year-old boy presents with a painful subgaleal mass and painful shoulder, and the following images are obtained (33A–C).
i. Where are the lesions located?
ii. Which additional dedicated scan of the brain should be performed in this disorder?
iii. What is the differential diagnosis of the bony lesions?

DIFFERENTIAL DIAGNOSIS Images 33D, E.

33 DIAGNOSIS Langerhans cell histiocytosis (LCH).

IMAGING FINDINGS Images 33A–C (scout image of the skull, sagittal contrast-enhanced T1, and CT scan of the scapula, respectively) demonstrate two lytic lesions of the skull and a destructive lesion of the left scapula. A round, well-defined lesion is seen in the left anterior parietal bone and another well-circumscribed but lobulated defect is visible in the right frontal bone. The postcontrast MR image reveals that the parietal defect is associated with an intensely enhancing soft tissue mass. A second destructive lytic bone lesion is visible in the left scapula, which expands the contour of the bone and may destroy cortex posteriorly (i,ii).

DIFFERENTIAL DIAGNOSIS The differential diagnosis (iii) of lytic skull lesion includes:
Multiple lesions
- Normal variant (e.g. parietal foramina) (33E, axial CT).
- Surgical defects (e.g. burr holes; shunt).
- Multiple myeloma (especially in patients >60 years old) (33D, skull radiograph).
- Metastases, lymphoma.
- Hyperparathyroidism.
- LCH (33A–C).
Solitary lesion
- Normal variant.
- Surgical defects (e.g. burr holes; shunt).
- Metastases, lymphoma, plasmacytoma.
- LCH.
- Ewings sarcoma.
- Lytic phase of Paget's disease.
- Osteomyelitis.
- Epidermoid.
- Haemangioma.
- Leptomeningeal cyst.
- Haemangiopericytoma (see Question 43).

When considering skull lesions, the differential should be based on an assessment of the number of lesions (single versus multiple) and the appearance of the lesion itself (margins, degree of bony destruction, internal matrix, and presence of a soft tissue mass). Clinical history (patient age or the presence of a known malignancy) might also influence the differential.

Image 33D shows multiple lytic skull lesions in a 70-year-old patient with multiple myeloma. Parietal foramina (33E) are a normal variant that are caused by emissary veins traversing the skull that join the sagittal sinus with external occipital venous branches; the smooth margins of these lesions and characteristic location should not be confused with pathology.

PATHOLOGY AND CLINICAL CORRELATION LCH is characterized by granulomas of Langerhans cell histiocytes involving any organ. The most common lesions of LCH are lytic skull defects and a pituitary stalk mass (which is associated with diabetes insipidus).

The classic lesion of LCH is described as having a beveled edge (with greater involvement of the inner table of the skull than the outer table). Rarely, LCH can be associated with geographic mastoid destruction, choroid plexus tumour, leptomeningeal nodules, and cerebellar white matter demyelination. Prognosis and therapeutic options depend upon symptoms, location, and extent of disease.

TEACHING PEARLS

➤ *For any lytic lesion of bone (particularly the skull or face) in a child, LCH should always be strongly considered.*
➤ *Lytic skull lesion and thick pituitary stalk in an infant or child are typical for histiocytosis.*
➤ *The skull is the most common bony site of LCH.*
➤ *Classic lesions have well-circumscribed margins with beveled edge and without marginal sclerosis. Lesions can show button seqestra in the healing phase.*
➤ *50% of bony lesions are polyostotic.*
➤ *Patients typically present before 2 years of age.*

34 A 29-year-old patient presents with nocturnal back pain. The following images are obtained (34A, B).
i. Name several primary osseous lesions commonly affecting the posterior elements.
ii. What is the central dense portion of this lesion called?
iii. What is the classic history for patients with this lesion?

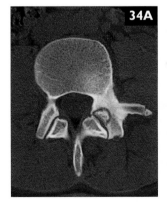 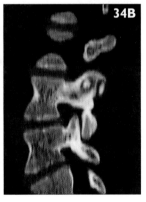

34: Answer

34 DIAGNOSIS Vertebral osteoid osteoma.

IMAGING FINDINGS There is a small intraosseous lesion within the left L3 inferior articulating facet seen on both axial and sagittally reconstructed CT images (**34A, B**). The lesion shows lucent periphery and a sclerotic central nidus.

DIFFERENTIAL DIAGNOSIS Primary osseous lesions of the posterior elements can be recalled with the pneumonic 'GO APE': giant cell tumour, osteoid osteoma/osteoblastoma, aneurismal bone cyst, plasmacytoma, and eosinophilic granuloma (hystiocytosis X) (**i**). In this case, the sclerotic nidus is classic for osteoid osteoma (**ii**). Metastatic disease is unlikely in a patient of this age.

PATHOLOGY AND CLINICAL CORRELATION Osteoid osteomas are benign bone-forming tumours. Twenty percent of these lesions are seen in the spine and 80% of the patients are less than 30 years old. They are similar to osteoblastomas and are primarily differentiated by size, with osteoid osteomas measuring less than 1.5 cm. The classic history is that of nocturnal pain relieved by nonsteroidal anti-inflammatory drugs (NSAIDs) (**iii**). When encountered in the spine, a scoliotic deformity can occur with concavity toward the side of the tumour. Visualization of the sclerotic nidus strongly suggests the diagnosis but can be difficult to appreciate on radiographs. For this reason, thin cut CT is the prefered imaging modality when osteoid osteoma of the spine is considered. When imaged with MRI, considerable surrounding marrow oedema can be seen. Treatment consists of surgical removal or radiofrequency ablation of the nidus.

TEACHING PEARLS
➤ *Osteoid osteomas are osseous lesions measuring less than 1.5 cm and showing a small sclerotic nidus.*
➤ *Osteoid osteoma is a cause of painful scoliosis in young patients.*
➤ *A history of focal nocturnal pain relieved by NSAIDs should raise suspicion for osteoid osteoma.*

REFERENCES
Ozaki T, *et al*. (2002). Osteoid osteoma and osteoblastoma of the spine: experiences with 22 Patients. *Clin Orthop Relat Res* **397**:394–402.
Yamamoto K, *et al*. (2005). Diagnostic efficacy of thin slice CT in osteoid osteoma of the thoracic spine: report of two cases. *J Spinal Disord Tech* **18**(2):182–4.

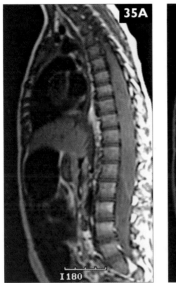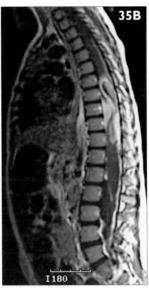

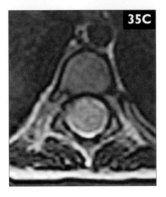

35 A 4-year-old girl presents with difficulty walking.
i. What are the imaging findings (35A–C)?
ii. Do appearances suggest a benign or malignant lesion?

35 DIAGNOSIS Glioblastoma multiforme of the cord.

IMAGING FINDINGS An intramedullary T2 hyperintense lesion of the thoracic cord is appreciated on all sequences (**35A**: sagittal T1-weighted; **35B**: sagittal T1-weighted (postcontrast); **35C**: axial T2-weighted). The thoracic cord shows marked expansion. There is strong, irregular enhancement of the mid thoracic cord (**35B**), with associated T2 hyperintensity (**35C**) (**i**). The combination of an expanded hyperintense cord with irregular enhancement is highly suggestive of a cord tumour.

PATHOLOGY, DIFFERENTIAL DIAGNOSIS, AND CLINICAL CORRELATION The majority of spinal cord tumours are primary neoplastic lesions, with secondary spread to the intramedullary spine a rare phenomenon. Spinal gliomas are the most common tumour in children, whereas in adults, ependymoma shows a slight predominance. The majority of glial cord tumours are benign astrocytomas (WHO grade 1 or 2), with more aggressive pathology, as seen in this case being more unusual (**ii**).

Presenting symptoms are frequently nonspecific, e.g. pain, gait or bladder difficulties and this may cause delay in diagnosis.

TEACHING PEARL
➤ *Primary intramedullary spinal tumours 'all' enhance, irrespective of grade.*

REFERENCE
Houten JK, Cooper PR (2000). Spinal cord astrocytomas: presentation, management, and outcome. *J Neuro Oncol* **47**(3):219–24.

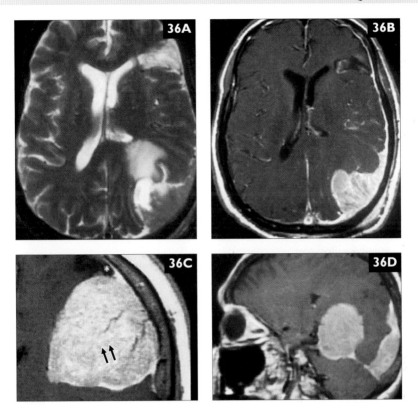

36 A 54-year-old male presents with headache and urinary symptoms, and the following images are obtained (36A, B).
i. Which sequences are shown?
ii. Describe the morphology, enhancement pattern, and extension of the lesions.
iii. What is the differential diagnosis for the bigger mass?

DIFFERENTIAL DIAGNOSIS Images 36C, D.

36 DIAGNOSIS Prostate metastasis.

IMAGING FINDINGS Images 36A, B (axial T2 and postcontrast axial T1, respectively) (i) demonstrate a T2 hyperintense, T1 hypointense wedge-shaped lesion in the inferior frontal gyrus consistent with an old infarct. More importantly, a heterogeneously enhancing extra-axial mass is seen in the left parieto-occipital region causing mass effect on the underlying brain parenchyma, with adjacent parenchymal oedema, effacement of the atrium of the left lateral ventricle, and midline shift to the right. The lesion is associated with extensive dural enhancement (extending around the entire left hemisphere). There is left-sided sulcal effacement (seen best on the T2-weighted image, compare with the right side) and leptomeningeal enhancement. In addition, there is a subgaleal component without frank destruction of the skull (ii).

DIFFERENTIAL DIAGNOSIS The differential diagnosis (iii) of a focal dural-based mass includes:

- Meningioma (36C, coronal contrast-enhanced T1).
- Lymphoma.
- Metastasis (prostate and breast) (36A, B).
- Plasmacytoma (36D, sagittal contrast-enhanced T1).
- Neurosarcoid (see Question 55).
- Tuberculosis.
- Pachymeningitis.
- Extramedullary haematopoiesis.
- Plus: see differential diagnosis of subdural lesion (Question 39).
- Plus: see differential diagnosis of localized leptomeningeal disease (see Question 41).
- Lymphoma, neurosarcoid, and TB can be multicompartmental.

The most common extra-axial mass is a meningioma. Image 36C demonstrates an intensely enhancing well-defined extra-axial mass adjacent to the left parietal lobe with a characteristic dural tail, intratumoural vessels (arrows), and hyperostosis, typical for common meningioma. Other neoplasms are a second, less likely consideration that might be raised in the correct clinical setting or when the imaging characteristics do not fit for a meningioma. Image 36D shows two large, enhancing lobular dural masses; biopsy revealed plasmacytoma, the solitary form of myeloma.

PATHOLOGY AND CLINICAL CORRELATION Meningeal metastases develop usually due to haematogenous spread from primary cancer. Patients present in 50% of cases with headache. Besides enhanced MR, lumbar puncture should be performed to make the diagnosis. Prognosis is dismal with a 1–2 months survival time in untreated malignant meningeal metastases. Survival can be improved up to 6–10 months by intrathecal and/or systemic chemotherapy and radiation of the entire neuraxis.

TEACHING PEARLS (CASE 36)
- ➤ *This differential diagnosis is a 'bread and butter' differential in neuroradiology: meningioma is by far the most common diagnosis.*
- ➤ *There are two types of meningeal metastases: dural and leptomeningeal metastases.*
- ➤ *Dural metastasis often resembles atypical, malignant meningioma or haemangiopericytoma.*
- ➤ *In children, medulloblastoma and leukaemia are the most common primaries.*
- ➤ *In adults, breast, lung, prostate, and melanoma are the most common primaries.*

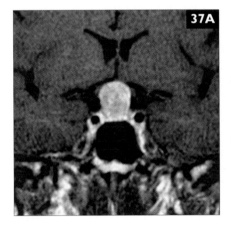 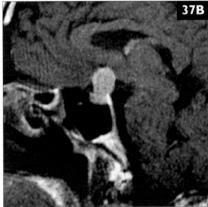

37 A 28-year-old postpartum female presents with headache, and the following images are obtained (**37A, B**).
i. Where is the abnormal enhancing mass centred?
ii. What pituitary abnormalities classically affect pregnant or postpartum females?
iii. What type of visual field defect is caused by inferior compression of the optic chiasm?

37 **DIAGNOSIS** Lymphocytic hypophysitis.

IMAGING FINDINGS Enhanced coronal T1 image (**37A**) shows a large mass centred within the sella turcica and showing suprasellar extension (**i**). The mass causes compression upon the optic chiasm superiorly. There is no lateral extension into the adjacent cavernous sinuses. Postcontrast sagittal image (**37B**) confirm the findings and shows intense enhancement homogeneously throughout the entire mass.

DIFFERENTIAL DIAGNOSIS The postpartum patient with pituitary abnormalities raises several possibilities. This population is predisposed to intrapituitary haemorrhage (Sheehan's syndrome) and lymphocytic hypophysitis (**ii**). Imaging findings could also represent a pituitary macroadenoma unrelated to the pregnancy.

PATHOLOGY AND CLINICAL CORRELATION Lymphocytic hypophysitis is an uncommon autoimmune disease primarily affecting women in the last 6 months of pregnancy or in the first 6 months postpartum. Infiltration of the anterior gland by lymphocytes, plasma cells, and macrophages usually inhibits pituitary function. Patients either present with symptoms related to pituitary dysfunction (most commonly amenorrhoea/galactorrhoea in women and sexual dysfunction in men) or from direct mass effect (headache, bilateral lateral [bitemporal] hemianopsia/tunnel vision due to optic chiasm compression) (**iii**).

Diagnosis is often difficult based on imaging findings. Classically, lymphocytic hypophysitis enhances diffusely, sometimes with a dural 'tail'. Pituitary haemorrhage may show regions on intrinsically increased T1 signal and decreased enhancement corresponding to blood products. Finally, adenomas generally show decreased or heterogeneous enhancement relative to the normal gland and tend to deviate the stalk from midline. However, definitive differentiation by imaging alone is impossible and diagnosis is confirmed by response to therapy or by biopsy.

The natural history of the disease is variable necessitating different therapeutic strategies. Since spontaneous remission can occur, close interval follow-up imaging is often performed in subclinical patients. In some cases, pituitary biopsy can be both diagnostic and therapeutic as recovery of glandular function can occur postprocedure. Surgical transphenoidal resection is performed when severe symptoms of compression are present. Recently, anti-inflammatory and immunosuppressive drugs have been suggested as treatment but their tong-term efficacy remains unproven.

TEACHING PEARLS
➤ *Lymphocytic hypophysitis primarily affects pregnant or postpartum females and is essentially indistinguishable from pituitary macroadenoma by imaging alone.*
➤ *Symptoms relate to pituitary dysfunction or mass effect.*
➤ *Subclinical cases are followed with the hope of spontaneous remission. Surgery is performed for severe compressive symptoms.*

REFERENCES (CASE 37)

Bellastella A, *et al.* (2003). Lymphocytic hypophysitis: a rare or underestimated disease? *Eur J Endocrinol* **149**:363–76.

Unluhizarci K, Bayram F, Colak R, *et al.* (2001). Distinct radiological and clinical appearance of lymphocytic hypophysitis. *J Clin Enocrinol Metab* **86**(5):1861–4.

(Images used courtesy of Elizabeth D. Ennis, MD, FACP.)

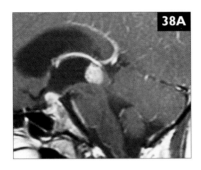

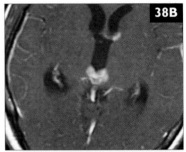

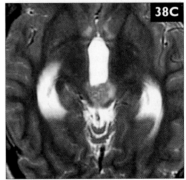

38 A patient presents and the following images are obtained (**38A–C**).

i. Where is the lesion located?

ii. What additional piece of demographic information is important to order the differential diagnosis?

38 DIAGNOSIS Germinoma.

IMAGING FINDINGS Images 38A–C (sagittal contrast-enhanced T1, axial contrast-enhanced T1, and axial contrast-enhanced T1, respectively) shows a heterogeneously enhancing mass which is isointense to the grey matter in T2. The mass engulfs the pineal gland and the 3rd ventricle (i). A second mass located at the left foramen of Munro with identical signal characteristics reflects CSF dissemination.

DIFFERENTIAL DIAGNOSIS The differential diagnosis for lesions occurring in the pineal gland include germ cell tumours (germinoma, teratoma, embryonal cell carcinoma, and choriocarcinoma), pineal cell tumours (pinealoblastoma, pineocytoma), pineal cyst, metastasis, meningioma, and tectal glioma. A key piece of information in formulating the differential diagnosis is the gender of the patient: 80% of lesions in men but only 50% of lesions in women will be germ cell tumours (ii).

PATHOLOGY AND CLINICAL CORRELATION Germinomas are germ cell tumours arising from primordial germ cells. Lesions have a propensity for the midline, occurring most commonly in the pineal gland and suprasellar region. Pineal gland germinomas are much more common in males (approximately 10:1). Patients are young, with the vast majority presenting before the age of 20. Symptoms depend on location. The lesion is malignant, but associated with excellent survival rates due to good response to radiation and chemotherapy. It is crucial to screen the entire neuraxis to evaluate for CSF dissemination.

TEACHING PEARLS
➤ *Pineal mass in men: 80% is germ cell tumour.*
➤ *Pineal mass in women: 50% is pineal cell tumour (pineocytoma or pineoblastoma) and 50% is germ cell tumour.*
➤ *Germinoma is the most common germ cell tumour (including teratoma, embryonal cell carcinoma, choriocarcinoma).*
➤ *Presentation depends on location. Pineal: Parinaud syndrome and/or headache to due hydrocephalus; suprasellar: diabetes insipidus and/or visual loss.*
➤ *It is a malignant tumour with a relatively benign prognosis due to radiation and chemotherapy sensitivity.*
➤ *The male : female ration is 10:1.*

REFERENCE
Veno T, *et al.* (2004). Spectrum of germ cell tumours: from head to toe. *Radiographics* 24:387–404.

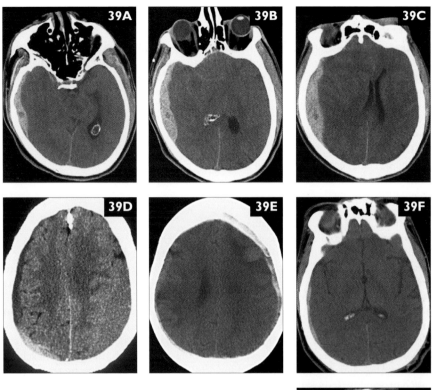

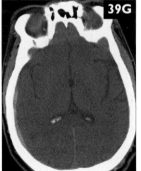

39 An 87-year-old male presents after a fall on the head, under anti-coagulant therapy. The following images are obtained (39A–C).

i. Where is the lesion localized in relation to the dura and what does the density tell you about the age of the lesion?

ii. What does the hypodense area within the lesion indicate?

iii. What other pathologies may occur in this location?

DIFFERENTIAL DIAGNOSIS Images 39D–G.

39 DIAGNOSIS Acute subdural haematoma (aSDH).

IMAGING FINDINGS Images 39A–C (axial unenhanced CT) demonstrate a hyperdense crescentic extra-axial collection, compatible with acute (ii) subdural haematoma (i). A hypodense focus within the haematoma is indicative of active extravasation in an anticoagulated patient (the 'swirl' sign). The subdural haematoma results in sulcal and ventricular effacement and severe midline shift to the left.

DIFFERENTIAL DIAGNOSIS The differential diagnosis (iii) of a subdural lesion includes:
• SDH (39A–C, D, F, G, axial NECT).
• Subdural empyema (see Question 44).
• Epidural haematoma.
• Subdural hygroma.
• Pachymeningitis.
• Motion artifact (39E, axial unenhanced CT).
• Plus: see differential diagnosis of focal dural-based mass (Question 36).
• Plus: see differential diagnosis of localized leptomeningeal disease (Question 41).
Image 39D from a child shows crescentic mixed SDH in the right hemisphere with anterior hypodense chronic portion and acute hyperdense portion posteriorly. Additionally, isodense lentiform SDH is seen adjacent to the left temporal and occipital lobes, raising suspicion of nonaccidental trauma. Image 39E is a motion artifact resembling hyperdense crescentic aSDH; the high density in this case actually represents the skull that is blurred by motion, although the true cause of this apparent abnormality should be clear from evaluation of the entire image. Image 39F (level 30, window 100) and 39G (level 80, window 200) are the same image presented with different window/level settings, demonstrating the importance of careful windowing in the detection of extra-axial haemorrhage, seen adjacent to the right temporal lobe in this case on 39G.

PATHOLOGY AND CLINICAL CORRELATION Acute SDH is defined as a '6-hour to 3-day-old crescent-shaped haemorrhagic collection between arachnoid and inner layer of dura, most common after trauma'. Haemorrhage comes from stretching and tearing of bridging cortical veins as they cross subdural space to drain into the dural sinus. The classic clinical description is of a 'lucid interval' of alertness after which the patient loses consciousness. Preoperative high-dose mannitol may improve poor outcome. The haemorrhage can extend over the entire hemisphere because the subdural space is continuous, interrupted only by the falx cerebri along the midline. Other important places to look for SDH are along the falx and along the tentorium cerebelli.

TEACHING PEARLS
➤ *NECT is the modality of choice for aSDH.*
➤ *Use a wide window setting (150–200 HU) to identify subtle SDH and avoid averaging with adjacent bone.*
➤ *Think of aSDH especially in patients with 'lucid' interval after trauma.*

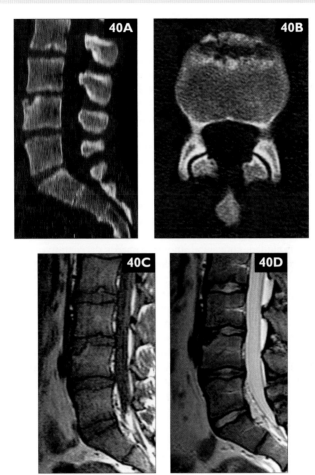

40 A 16-year-old child presents with back pain. The following images are obtained (40A–D).

i. Is there an acute fracture involving the superior L4 endplate?
ii. What is the most sensitive MR sequence to evaluate for acute fracture?
iii. What is a Schmorl's node?

40 DIAGNOSIS Limbus vertebra.

IMAGING FINDINGS Sagittal and axial CT demonstrate irregularity of the anterior superior L4 endplate (**40A, B**). There is focal anterior wedging and a small separate bone fragment anterior to the defect. A second central inferior endplate irregularity is seen at L2. Sagittal MRI images confirm the findings and show no abnormal marrow signal on T1 images (**40C**). T2 images show hypointense disc material herniating into the endplate defects (**40D**).

DIFFERENTIAL DIAGNOSIS While any endplate irregularity can mimic a fracture, the fact that there is no abnormal marrow signal definitively excludes the possibility of acute fracture (**i**). Though not shown in this case, inversion recovery (STIR) images are most sensitive in evaluating for acute fracture (**ii**). Increased signal intensity corresponds to marrow oedema with fracture. Almost as good are T1 sequences, in which marrow oedema would appear dark.

As fracture is excluded, congenital anomaly and/or degenerative changes are most likely. T2 images help by demonstrating low signal disc material herniating into the endplate defects. This is consistent with degenerative disc change. The L4 abnormality is a classic example of a limbus vertebra. The endplate irregularity at L2 represents a small Schmorl's node. The aetiology of both lesions is similar and they are often seen together.

PATHOLOGY AND CLINICAL CORRELATION Limbus vertebra and Schmorl's nodes are (with Scheuermann's disease) part of a spectrum of endplate irregularities seen rather commonly in childhood. Indeed, the incidence of all three processes appears to be on the rise but this may simply relate to increased utilization of imaging. The exact aetiology is uncertain, but an event or process triggers degenerative changes including loss of disc height and water content (resulting in dark disc material on T2 images), as well as vertebral body endplate irregularity and structural weakness.

A Schmorl's node occurs when disc material herniates into a weakened endplate (**iii**). A limbus vertebra can be thought of as a subset of Schmorl's nodes in which the herniation occurs near the endplate margin and undermines the ring epiphysis. This separates the epiphyseal ossification centre from the vertebral body proper and accounts for the abnormal anterior calcification seen in this case. Scheuermann's disease is the result of multiple tiny endplate irregularities and small associated herniations on both adjacent endplates resulting in a markedly irregular disc space. All three entities are variable in clinical significance. For incompletely understood reasons, some patients have pain related to these changes while the majority do not.

TEACHING PEARLS
➤ *Evaluation of marrow signal on STIR and/or T1 sequences helps confirm or exclude acute fractures.*
➤ *Limbus vertebra, Schmorl's nodes, and Scheuermann's disease are a spectrum of disease all resulting from degenerative endplate changes during childhood.*

REFERENCES (CASE 40)

Goldman AB, Ghelman B, Doherty J (1990). Posterior limbus vertebrae: a cause of radiating back pain in adolescents and young adults. *Skeletal Radiol* **19**(7):501–7.

Swischuk LE, John SD, Allberty S (1998). Disc degenerative disease in childhood: Scheuermann's disease, Schmorl's nodes, and limbus vertebra: MRI findings in 12 patients. *Pediatr Radiol* **28**:334–8.

Yagan R (1984). CT diagnosis of limbus vertebra. *J Comput Assist Tomogr* **8**(1):149–51.

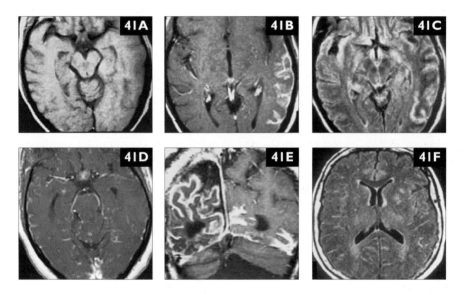

41 A 45-year-old female with headache and known breast cancer presents, and the following images are obtained (**41A–C**).

i. Which sequences are shown?

ii. Which structures of the brain are affected by this disease process?

iii. What is the most common origin of the lesion in children and adults?

DIFFERENTIAL DIAGNOSIS Images 41D–F.

41 **DIAGNOSIS** Carcinomatous meningitis.

IMAGING FINDINGS Images 41A–C (axial T1, axial contrast-enhanced T1, and axial FLAIR, respectively) (i) demonstrate leptomeningeal enhancement and hyperintense cerebrospinal fluid (CSF) in the sulci of the left temporal lobe (ii), compatible with carcinomatous meningitis. Note that the normal CSF on the FLAIR image (41C) is black, while the CSF over the left temporal lobe is increased in signal; this is an important abnormality to detect on FLAIR images.

DIFFERENTIAL DIAGNOSIS The differential diagnosis of a localized leptomeningeal disease includes:
- Infectious meningitis.
- Carcinomatous meningitis (41A–C).
- Tuberculosis (TB) (see Question 47).
- Sarcoidosis (41D, axial contrast-enhanced T1).
- Sturge–Weber syndrome (41E, coronal contrast-enhanced T1).
- Coccidioidomycosis (41F, axial FLAIR).
- Plus: see differential diagnosis of focal dural-based tumour (Question 36).
- Plus: see differential diagnosis of subdural lesion (Question 39).

Forming a differential diagnosis first requires precisely localizing the abnormality: in this case, there is leptomeningeal enhancement, which we can confirm because the enhancement follows the gyral contours and fills the sulci. Broad differential categories for leptomeningeal enhancement include infection, neoplasm (carcinomatous meningitis), and inflammation. Generally, carcinomatous meningitis will have a more nodular configuration, although this is not very apparent in the current case.

Image 41D (sarcoidosis) shows leptomeningeal enhancement; notice the thin enhancement that follows gyral contours and outlines the sulci. Image 41 depicts Sturge–Weber syndrome with right hemisphere atrophy, bilateral (right greater than left) leptomeningeal enhancement due to pial angiomatosis, and dural thickening (both at the falx cerebri and tentorium). Image 41 is an example of coccidioidomycosis with brain oedema and meningitis.

PATHOLOGY AND CLINICAL CORRELATION Carcinomatous meningitis (leptomeningeal metastases) is more common than dural metastases (see Question 36); however, the two may coexist. Carcinomatous meningitis usually develops due to haematogenous spread from primary cancer. Patients present in 50% of cases with headache. Besides enhanced MR, lumbar puncture should be performed to make the diagnosis. Prognosis is dismal, with a 1–2 months survival time in untreated malignant meningeal metastases. Survival can be improved up to 6–10 months by intrathecal and/or systemic chemotherapy and radiation of the entire neuraxis.

TEACHING PEARLS (CASE 41)

➤ *For focal leptomeningeal disease, consider TB at the skull base and carcinomatosis at the convexities.*

➤ *Meninges are hyperintense and thickened. CSF in the sulci does not null on FLAIR.*

➤ *Leptomeninges insinuate into cerebral sulci, which is a sign that helps to distinguish a leptomeningeal process from a dural one.*

➤ *Carcinomatosis occurs in up to 25% of all cancer patients.*

➤ *The most common primary tumours in children are medulloblastoma and leukaemia; in adults are breast, small-cell lung cancer, gastric, ovary, melanoma, lymphoma/leukaemia (iii).*

➤ *MRI is more sensitive than CT.*

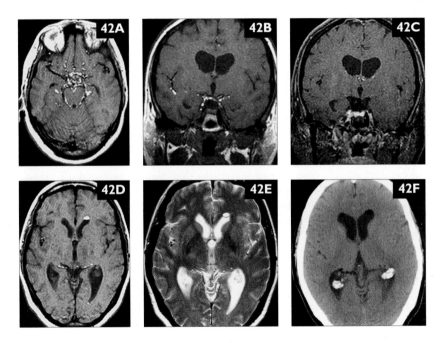

42 A 30-year-old patient presents with acute onset headache. The following images are obtained (**42A–F**).

i. Is the abnormal signal intra- or extra-axial?

ii. What types of substances are bright on T1-weighted images?

iii.Why is the abnormality no longer apparent on **42C** (obtained at the same time as the similar coronal slice in **42B**)?

42 DIAGNOSIS Ruptured dermoid.

IMAGING FINDINGS On unenhanced T1-weighted axial (**42A,D**) and coronal (**42B**) images, there are multifocal regions of extra-axial hyperintensity within the subarachnoid space primarily at the basilar cisterns (**i**). These hyperintensities are no longer apparent on fat-suppressed T1 coronal image (**42C**). Abnormal signal appears to 'float' within the nondependent lateral ventricles and is bright on T2 (**42E**) and extremely dark on unenhanced CT (**42F**).

DIFFERENTIAL DIAGNOSIS Few things are bright on unenhanced T1-weighted images. Among the most common are fat/lipid, subacute blood products, and extremely protinaceous material (**ii**). In this case, increased T1 signal spread throughout the subarachnoid space should immediately raise concern for ruptured dermoid with diffuse spread of lipid material. The diagnosis is confirmed by the reduction in signal on the fat-suppressed images (**iii**). Findings correlate with low density and negative Houndsfeld units on the accompanying CT scan.

PATHOLOGY AND CLINICAL CORRELATION The embryology of dermoid cysts is commonly misunderstood. Epidermoids and dermoids are very similar, both arising entirely from trapped ectodermal cell rests. Epidermoids contain squamous epithelium only. Dermoids contain squamous epithelium in addition to hair and sebaceous and sweat glands. Teratomas, on the other hand, are true neoplasms arising from misplaced embryologic germ cells and often contain at least two of the three embryonic germ layers (**ii**). It is felt that intracranial dermoids arise from embryological accidents that occur earlier than similar events leading to epidermoid cysts. This may explain the near midline location of dermoids. On imaging, it is the lipid product of sebaceous gland secretions that shows increased T1 signal in dermoids rather than mesodermal adipose.

Dermoids represent 0.04–0.25% of intracranial neoplasms and are four to 10 times less common than epidermoids. Dermoids show slow growth due to accumulation of squamous and sebaceous products. Complications include: mass effect upon adjacent structures, spinal dysraphism (if posterior or within the spinal canal), infection (if associated with a sinus tract), and rupture (**iii**). Most ruptures are spontaneous but they can be precipitated by trauma. Initially felt to be universally fatal, it is now known that ruptured dermoids can have varied presentations and outcome. The most common presenting symptoms include headache, seizure, temporary sensory or motor hemisyndrome, and chemical meningitis. Treatment for rupture is usually supportive. Rarely, surgical evacuation and irrigation of the CSF spaces is attempted.

TEACHING PEARLS
➤ *Fat/lipid, subacute blood, and highly proteinaceous substances are bright on T1-weighted images.*
➤ *Ruptures dermoid cysts cause disseminated T1 hyperintensity throughout the subarachnoid space.*
➤ *Dermoids and epidermoids are ectodermal inclusion cysts. Teratomas are true neoplasms arising from at least two of the three embryonic germ layers.*

REFERENCES
Smirniotopoulos J, Chiechi M (1995). Teratomas, dermoids, and epidermoids of the head and neck. *Radiographics* 15:1437–55.
Stendel R, *et al.* (2002). Ruptured intracranial dermoid cysts. *Surg Neurol* 57:391–8.

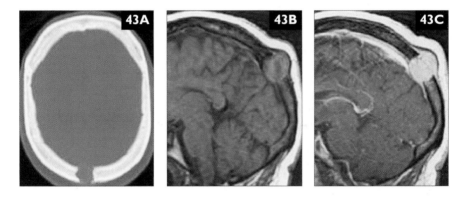

43 A 48-year-old male presents with a growing lump over the occiput. The following images are obtained (43A–C).
i. What is the abnormality? Where is it located?
ii. What is the most likely diagnosis?

43 **DIAGNOSIS** Haemangiopericytoma.

IMAGING FINDINGS Images 43A–C (axial CT, sagittal T1, and contrast-enhanced sagittal T1, respectively) show a vividly enhancing dural based mass that traverses the skull at the junction of the sagittal and lambdoid sutures, extending into the subgaleal space (i). It is important to note that this is a rare presentation of a rare tumour.

DIFFERENTIAL DIAGNOSIS This large lesion has a broad differential diagnosis based on the intersection of two different differential diagnoses, specifically, (1) lytic skull lesions in an adult, and (2) pachymeningeal or dural based lesions. The most likely is dural metastasis or plasmacytoma with calvarial invasion. Meningioma and its variants, such as hemangiopericytomas, are also extra-axial and may be difficult to differentiate from other homogeneously enhancing dural masses, although meningioma is more commonly associated with hyperostosis. Lymphoma, neuro-sarcoidosis, tuberculosis, or other potential causes of pachymeningeal thickening are less likely to have this pattern of osseous involvement. The entity pictured here is hemangiopericytoma (ii).

PATHOLOGY AND CLINICAL CORRELATION Hemangiopericytoma is a sarcoma arising from pericytes, contractile mesenchymal cells associated with capillaries. The lesion most commonly occurs in the lower extremities, pelvis, and retroperitoneum, but 15% occur in the head and neck region. An enhancing extra-axial mass with dural involvement, heterogeneous enhancement, and possible osseous involvement is typical. Hemangiopericytoma should be considered when a lesion resembles a meningioma but there are atypical features.

TEACHING PEARLS
➤ *Consider haemangiopericytoma in a meningioma-like mass with atypical features like bone destruction and extensive surrounding oedema, but without calcification or hyperostosis.*
➤ *It is a lobular, heterogenously enhancing highly vascular WHO grade 2 or 3 extra-axial tumour.*
➤ *Extracranial metastases occur in up to 30% and local recurrence is common.*
➤ *It is most common in 40–60-year-old adults.*

REFERENCE
Chiechi MV, *et al.* (1996). Intracranial hemangiopericytomas: MR and CT features. *AJNR* 17:1365–71.

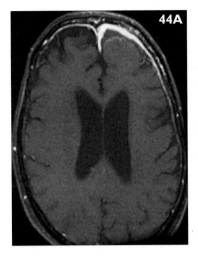

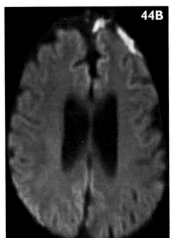

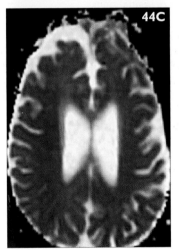

44 A 34-year-old male presents with fever and headaches. The patient reports a history of sinusitis. Images (44A–C) are obtained.
i. Where is the abnormality located?
ii. What are the images presented, and how do they help narrow the differential diagnosis?

44 DIAGNOSIS   Subdural empyema (SDE).

IMAGING FINDINGS   Images 44A–C (contrast-enhanced axial T1, DWI, and ADC, respectively) demonstrate a crescentic, intensely enhancing extra-axial process located adjacent to both frontal lobes, more on the left; the extension along the falx suggests a subdural location (**i**). The DWI map shows that this collection has restricted diffusion (bright areas) confirmed by the ADC map (dark areas), consistent with infection (**ii**).

DIFFERENTIAL DIAGNOSIS   Differential diagnosis includes any subdural process, such as SDE or subdural haematoma. Subdural collections that would mimic CSF signal (such as subdural hygroma or subdural effusion) are excluded. Although the restricted diffusion suggests an infected collection, certain stages of haemorrhagic clot can have a similar appearance on DWI/ADC maps, so that the clinical history becomes crucial in distinguishing these processes. A dural compartment based mass (as opposed to subdural) is less likely, given the involvement deep to the dural reflection of the anterior margin of the superior sagittal sinus.

PATHOLOGY AND CLINICAL CORRELATION   SDE is an extra-axial, rim-enhancing fluid collection, most commonly located over the convexity or along the midline. This can either be associated with superinfection by concurrent meningitis (in infants and small children), or, more commonly, with paranasal sinus disease (in older children and adults). In the latter case, there is usually direct spread from the posterior wall of the frontal sinus. SDE is a neurosurgical emergency and can be fatal if not recognized. CSF fluid analysis can be normal. Complications include cerebritis and venous thrombosis.

TEACHING PEARLS
- *Gadolinium-enhanced MR (vivid, often rim enhancement) with DWI (restricted diffusion) is more sensitive and specific than CT.*
- *Chronic subdural haematoma might be indistinguishable: remember that certain stages of haemorrhage can also appear to have restricted diffusion.*
- *Epidural empyema is biconvex with displacement of dura from the inner table of skull.*
- *Consider empyema in a patient with neurological symptoms, sinusitis, and frontal subgaleal abscess ('Pott´s puffy tumour').*
- *SDE is a neurosurgical emergency.*

REFERENCES
Rich PM, Deasy NP, Jarosz JM (2000). Intracranial dural empyema. *BJR* 73:1329–36.
Zimmerman RD, Leeds NE, Danziger A (1984). Subdural empyema: CT findings. *Radiology* 150:417–22.

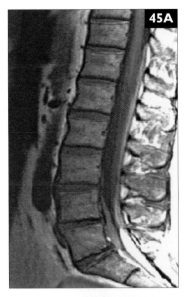
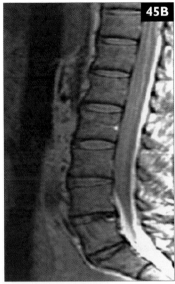
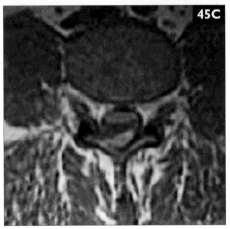

45 A 51-year-old male patient is admitted with head trauma and low back pain, and the following images are obtained (45A–C).
i. What findings are seen?
ii. What are the differential diagnoses?

45 DIAGNOSIS Epidural haematoma.

IMAGING FINDINGS The images show tapered ventral and dorsal epidural collections, showing iso/ hyperintensity on T1-weighted imaging and hyperintensity on T2-weighted imaging, with compression of the thecal sac and cauda equina (i).

DIFFERENTIAL DIAGNOSIS While signal characteristics and history are most in keeping with epidural haematoma, the differential would include epidural abscess, epidural lipomatosis, and subdural haematoma (ii).

PATHOLOGY AND CLINICAL CORRELATION Predisposing factors for epidural haematoma include surgery, prior attempts at lumbar puncture, epidural anesthesia, trauma, anticoagulation, and underlying vascular lesions. Haemorrhage occurs from the epidural venous plexus and is most commonly seen in the cervical and thoracic regions, where lesions commonly extend over multiple levels.

TEACHING PEARL
➤ *Epidural haematoma may be asymptomatic, extending over multiple levels without compromising the thecal sac.*

REFERENCE
Boukobza M, *et al.* (1994). Spinal epidural haematoma: report of 11 cases and review of the literature. *Neuroradiology* 36(6):456–9.

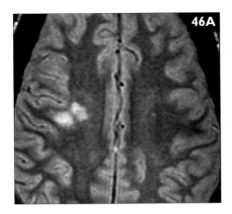

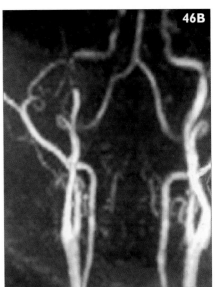

46 A 29-year-old male presents with acute onset neurological changes suggestive of an infarct. He reports a recent car accident in which he was a restrained passenger.
i. Which sequences are shown (46A–C)?
ii. What clinical situations should prompt suspicion for this diagnosis?

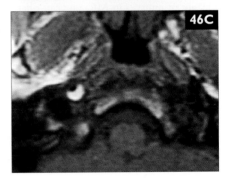

46 DIAGNOSIS Extracranial internal carotid artery (ICA) dissection.

IMAGING FINDINGS Image **46A** (FLAIR) shows hyperintense signal in the right hemispheric subcortical white matter (WM) and centrum semiovale, representing an infarct. Image **46B** (3D TOF unenhanced MRA) depicts marked, tapered narrowing of the right distal extracranial ICA as it enters the skull base, secondary to dissection. Axial T1-weighted image with fat saturation ('fatsat') in **46C** reveals crescentic hyperintense signal adjacent to a narrowed right ICA flow void, consistent with the subacute T1-bright met-haemoglobin stage of haemorrhage, suggesting extracranial dissection (i).

DIFFERENTIAL DIAGNOSIS The differential diagnosis of focal T2 hyperintense WM lesions is broad, and includes infarct, demyelination, trauma (specifically diffuse axonal injury, DAI), and tumour. The acuity of symptom/lesion onset aids in narrowing this differential (e.g. infarct = acute, demyelination = subacute, tumour = chronic).

PATHOLOGY AND CLINICAL CORRELATION Extracranial ICA dissection is a haemorrhagic tear within the vessel wall, often spontaneous, occasionally related to heavy exertion such as weight-lifting. The abnormality can be detected either by directly visualizing the dissection flap, or by identifying alterations in the calibre and appearance of the vessel at the site of injury. On MR, one can often see a crescentic intramural haematoma at the region of the flap, with tapered narrowing ('string-sign') and diminished flow related signal. An abrupt 'step off' is typically noted at the site of calibre change. Occlusion is common but resolves in 90% of cases with appropriate long-term anticoagulation therapy. Pseudoaneurysm is a less common and often more serious complication, and resolves in only roughly 50% of appropriately treated cases. High quality 'fatsat T1' imaging is necessary to visualize the hyperintense crescentic intramural haematoma, but as this reflects the subacute met-haemoglobin stage of haemorrhage, this sign is a *specific* but not a *sensitive* indicator of dissection. Most common location for extracranial dissection is in the ICA between the skull base and a point several centimetres cranial to the carotid bifurcation, and the second most common location is the vertebral artery at the C1–C2 level. No parenchymal changes are seen unless there is secondary infarct in the vascular territory of the affected vessel.

TEACHING PEARLS
- *High suspicion is necessary in order to acquire the appropriate imaging (CT angiography or MR angiography); sometimes neck pain may be the only presenting complaint.*
- *Consider dissection in a young or middle-aged adult with stroke and unrelenting head or neck ache (ii).*
- *CTA may be helpful acutely; T1-fat suppressed imaging is specific but not sensitive and may not be positive in the acute setting.*

REFERENCES (CASE 46)
Beletsky V, Norris JW (2001). Spontaneous dissection of the carotid and vertebral arteries. *N Engl J Med* **345**(6):467.
Fisher CM, Ojemann RG, Roberson GH (1978). Spontaneous dissection of cervico-cerebral arteries. *Can J Neurol Sci* **5**(1):9–19.
Stallmayer MJ, *et al.* (2006). Imaging of traumatic neurovascular injury. *Radiol Clin North Am* **44**:13–39.

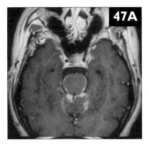
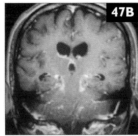
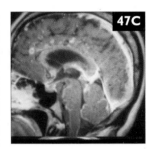

47 A 35-year-old male presents with fevers and meningeal signs. CSF analysis after lumbar puncture reveals increased protein, low glucose, and lymphocytes, although no organism is identified. Images are obtained (47A–C).
i. Which sequences are shown?
ii. Which structures of the brain are affected by this disease process?

48 A 60-year-old male patient presents with back pain, and the following images are obtained (48A, B).
i. Describe the abnormality seen at the L5/S1 level.
ii. What do you think the composition of the lesion is?
iii. Where do you think it is arising from?

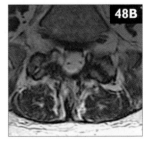

47 **Diagnosis** Tuberculosis (TB).

Imaging findings Images **47A–C** (axial, coronal, and sagittal contrast-enhanced T1, respectively) (i) show intense enhancement of the basal meninges, particularly adjacent to the inferior surface of frontal lobe, along the floor of the 3rd ventricle, and coating the brainstem and cerebellum (ii).

Differential diagnosis The key feature is the leptomeningeal compartmentalization of the abnormality, predominantly at the skull base, with sulcal (aka pial, aka subarachnoid space) enhancement. The differential diagnosis of localized leptomeningeal disease includes carcinomatous meningitis, infectious meningitis, TB, lymphoma/sarcoidosis (as per the discussion of Question 55), or connective tissue disorders such as RA or SLE.

Pathology and clinical correlation TB must always be considered if there is leptomeningeal enhancement at the skull base (basal meningitis). CSF analysis must include specific staining and culture in search of acid-fast bacilli. Tuberculomas are intraparenchymal lesions, most commonly supratentorial and multiple. CNS infection is caused by haematogenous spread of infection from another location (such as the lungs). TB is a much more common CNS abnormality in the developing world. Clinical presentation is highly variable. Morbidity is seen in 80% of cases and is fatal in 25–30% of cases.

Teaching pearls
> *Think of TB in a patient with both meningitis and parenchymal lesions.*
> *Meningitis shows typically basilar prominence, marked meningeal enhancement, and increased intensity of the basal cisterns on FLAIR sequences due to proteinaceous exudate.*
> *Parenchymal lesions (tuberculomas) are solid or ring-enhancing and often seen in the parietal lobes.*

Reference
Shah GV (2000). Central nervous system tuberculosis: imaging manifestations. *Neuroimaging Clin N Am* **10**:355–74.

48 Diagnosis Right facet joint synovial cyst.

Imaging findings A cystic lesion (**ii**) is seen arising from the anterior aspect of the right L5/S1 facet joint (**iii**), which shows underlying degenerative changes. It indents the right aspect of the thecal sac (**i**).

Pathology and clinical correlation Synovial cysts are most commonly seen at L4/L5 or L5/S1 and arise secondary to facet degeneration. On MR, they commonly show a signal intensity similar to cerebrospinal fluid, although they may be slightly hyperintense on T1-weighted imaging. Occasionally, cysts may show haemorrhage, resulting in a low signal intensity on T2-weighted imaging. The cyst periphery may enhance with contrast or may show calcification (best seen on CT). Their clinical importance is that they may cause compression of the thecal sac which, if severe, or associated with other degenerative changes, may cause canal stenosis.

Teaching pearl
➤ *Synovial cysts may be a cause of canal stenosis.*

Reference
Liu SS, *et al.* (1990). Synovial cysts of the lumbosacral spine: diagnosis by MR imaging. *Am J Roentgenol* **154**(1):163–166.

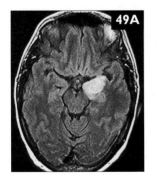 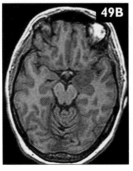 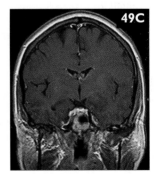

49 A 37-year-old patient presents with new-onset seizures, and the following images are obtained (**49A–C**).
i. What lobe is affected by this signal abnormality?
ii. Which viral encephalitis is predisposed to affect the medial temporal lobes?
iii. The term 'low-grade' typically refers to tumours of which WHO grades?

49 DIAGNOSIS Low-grade astrocytoma (WHO grade 2).

IMAGING FINDINGS There is focal increased T2/FLAIR signal seen within the anterior medial left temporal lobe (**49A**) (**i**). This corresponds to hypointense T1 signal (**49B**) and shows no contrast enhancement (**49C**). No surrounding vasogenic oedema is seen. There is very little mass effect and no volume loss. No other lesions were seen.

DIFFERENTIAL DIAGNOSIS Primary differential diagnosis includes low-grade primary glial tumour, encephalitis, and infarction. Of the infectious causes, herpes encephalitis is the most worrisome and should always be considered when medial temporal abnormality is present (**ii**). Indeed, it is common to treat the patient empirically with anti-viral medication until serology and CSF studies can be definitively evaluated. The lack of diffusion restriction essentially rules out infarction. Metastatic disease is not seriously considered due to the lack of enhancement.

PATHOLOGY AND CLINICAL CORRELATION Low-grade astrocytomas (WHO grade 1 and 2) can be either focal of diffuse (**iii**). When focal, they can appear extremely benign. Though usually absent, minimal enhancement can occasionally be seen. Pathologically, all astrocytomas originate within white matter but these tumours can extend into the grey matter of the cortex or deep nuclei. Neoplastic cells can extend beyond the margins of MR signal abnormality. More worrisome, these tumours have the potential for malignant progression into anaplastic astrocytomas. Indeed, most cases of postresection recurrence are due to dedifferentiation.

Low-grade astrocytomas represent approximately 25% of all glial tumours. Presentation depends on the area of the brain involved. Approximately 2/3 of lesions are supratentorial while the remaining 1/3 are seen in the cerebellum and brainstem. Though they can affect any age group, patients tend to be younger than those affected by glioblastoma multiforme (WHO grade 4). Treatment is surgical resection. Adjuvant chemo- and radiation therapy is also often administered.

TEACHING PEARLS
➢ *Low-grade astrocytomas can be either focal or diffuse.*
➢ *The lack of enhancement and surrounding oedema can make these lesions appear extremely benign.*
➢ *Neoplastic cells extend beyond the margins of signal abnormality.*

REFERENCES
Burger PC, Scheithauer BW, Vogel FS (2002). *Surgical Pathology of the Nervous System and its Coverings.* The Brain: Tumours. 4th edn. Churchill Livingstone, Philadelphia, pp. 160–77.
Kleihues P, Cavenee WK (2000). *Pathology and Genetics of Tumours of the Nervous System.* Diffuse astrocytoma. IARC Press, Lyon, pp. 22–6.
Osborn AG, *et al.* (2004). Brain. Diffuse astrocytoma, low-grade. *AMIRSYS*, Salt Lake City, I–6 pp.8–11.
Wessels PH, *et al.*(2003). Supratentorial grade II astrocytoma: biological features and clinical course. *Lancet Neurol* 2(7):395–403.

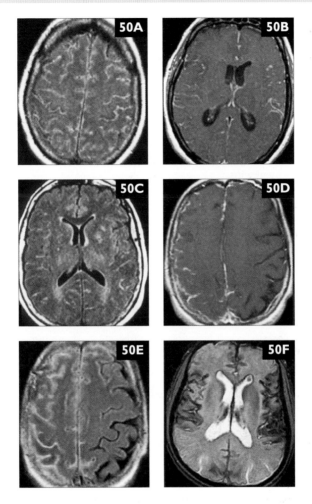

50 A 23-year-old female presents with headache, fever, nuchal rigidity, and altered mental status. The following images are obtained (50A, B).
i. Which sequences are shown?
ii. What is the pathological finding?
iii. What are typical complications of this disorder?
iv. What is the differential diagnosis?

DIFFERENTIAL DIAGNOSIS Images 50C–F.

50 **Diagnosis** Pneumococcal meningitis.

Imaging findings Images 50A, B (axial FLAIR, axial contrast-enhanced T1, respectively) (i) show hyperintensity and enhancement in the sulci and cisterns, representing exudate in a patient with pneumococcus meningitis (ii).

Differential diagnosis The differential diagnosis (iv) of a diffuse leptomeningeal disease includes:
- Bacterial meningitis (e.g. *S. pneumoniae*) (50A, B)
- Viral meningitis.
- Carcinomatous meningitis.
- Neurosarcoid.
- Fungal meningitis (e.g. coccidiomycosis) (50C, axial FLAIR).
- Rheumatoid meningitis (50D, E, axial contrast-enhanced T1 and FLAIR).
- Plus: see differential diagnosis for localized leptomeningeal disease (Question 33).
Mimics:
- Increased FLAIR signal in cerebrospinal fluid (CSF):
  - Subarachnoid haemorrhage.
  - 100% inspired oxygen.
  - Acute stroke (parenchymal oedema, congestion).
  - Gadolinium in CSF (dialysis-dependent patient).
  - Artifact.
- Superficial haemosiderosis (50F, T2*GRE).
- Moyamoya (see Question 74).

Pathology and clinical correlation Meningitis is defined as inflammatory infiltration of the pia mater, arachnoid, and CSF, most commonly caused by haematogenous dissemination from a distant infection. Fungal and tuberculous meningitis are often basilar, nodular, and confluent. Meningitis is associated with three major types of complications; impaired CSF resorption may cause extraventricular obstructive hydrocephalus with increased intracranial pressure and perfusion alterations. Complications include empyema, ventriculitis, abscess, and vascular complications including ischaemia due to arterial spasm or infectious arteritis (iii).

Teaching pearls
➤ *Imaging may be normal early in the disease process.*
➤ *Imaging findings are nonspecific, with intense leptomeningeal enhancement on contrast-enhanced T1 and hyperintense signal in sulci and cisterns on FLAIR and DWI sequences.*
➤ *Imaging delineates complications that occur in about 50% of adult patients.*
➤ *Despite effective anti-microbial agents, overall mortality rate is still 25%.*

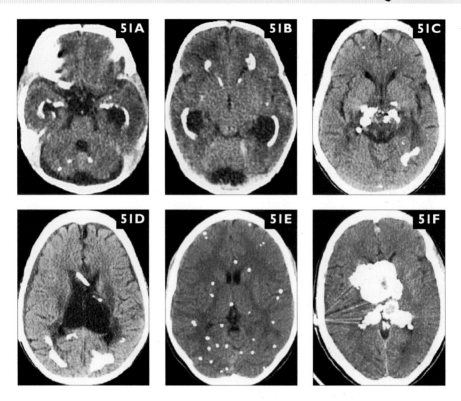

51 A 6-month-old male newborn presents with microcephaly and hearing loss. The following images are obtained (51A–D).

i. What do the hyperdensities represent and where are they localized?

ii. What other cerebral and cerebellar pathologies would you expect in this disorder?

iii. What modality is usually used for neonatal screening?

iv. What is the differential diagnosis?

DIFFERENTIAL DIAGNOSIS Images 51E, F.

51 Diagnosis Congenital cytomegalovirus (CMV).

Imaging findings Images **51A–D** (axial unenhanced CT) demonstrate multifocal coarse periventricular and subependymal calcifications involving the periventricular white matter (WM) (**51A, B**), the cerebellum (**51A**), the occipital lobe (**51D**) and deep grey nuclei (**51C**) (**i**). Dilation of the lateral ventricle (especially the body, atrium, and temporal horn) due to WM volume loss is best seen on **51D**.

Differential diagnosis The differential diagnosis (**iv**) of periventricular calcification includes:
In neonates:
• CMV (**51A–D**, axial NECT).
• Toxoplasmosis.
• Congenital HIV.
• Lymphocytic choriomeningitis (LCM).
• Rubella virus.
In any age-group:
• Tuberous sclerosis (see Question **13**).
Additional causes of parenchymal calcifications (not periventricular in distribution) are shown in images **51E, F**. Image **51E** demonstrates nodular calcified stage of neurocysticercosis with multiple calcified shrunken nodules in both hemispheres. Image **51F** demonstrates an intensely calcified midline meningioma localized in the body, atrium, and septum pellucidum of the lateral ventricle bilaterally with extraventricular extension.

Pathology and clinical correlation Congenital CMV infection is caused by transplacental transmission. Cranial sonography is used for neonatal screening (**iii**). Most newborns with central nervous system (CNS) involvement have major neurodevelopmental sequelae.

Teaching pearls
➢ *CMV is the most common intrauterine infection affecting 1% of all newborns.*
➢ *It presents with microcephaly, periventricular calcifications, cortical gyral abnormalities, and cerebellar hypoplasia (ii).*
➢ *Clinically, think of CMV in a microcephalic, developmentally delayed infant with sensorineural hearing loss (SNHL).*
➢ *However, most infected newborns appear normal.*

References
Abe K, *et al.* (2004). Comparison of conventional and diffusion-weighted MRI and proton MR spectroscopy in patients with mitochondrial encephalomyopathy, lactic acidosis, and stroke-like events. *Neuroradiology* 46(2):113–7.
Osborn AG, *et al.* (2004). *Brain.* Amirsys, Salt Lake City, Chapter I-10, pp. 28–31.

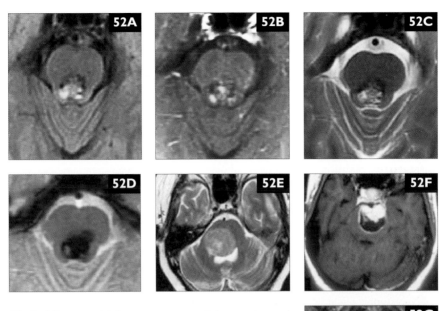

52 A 15-year-old boy presents with ataxia and headache, and the following images are obtained (52A–D).
i. What makes the rim of the mass in 52C hypointense?
ii. Which sequence is shown in 52D and what can you conclude from it?
iii. What other disorders typically can occur in this location?

DIFFERENTIAL DIAGNOSIS Images 52E–G.

52 **Diagnosis** Cavernous malformation (CM).

Imaging findings Images 52A–D (axial T1, axial T1 postgadolinium, axial T2, axial gradient echo, respectively) demonstrate a CM in the posterior pons compressing the 4th ventricle. The mass demonstrates no significant enhancement (compare **52A** and **52B**). Mixed signal characteristics suggest blood products in different stages of evolution, surrounded by a rim of hypointense hemosiderin (**i**) that causes susceptibility artifact on the gradient echo image shown in **52D** (**ii**). No oedema or mass effect is visible.

Differential diagnosis The differential diagnosis (**iii**) of a brainstem mass includes:
• Metastasis (**52F**; axial T1 postgadolinium).
• Pontine glioma (**52E**; axial T2).
• Pontine infarct.
• Multiple sclerosis/ acute disseminated encephalomyelitis.
• CM (**52A–D**).
• Neurofibromatosis type 1.
• Osmotic demyelination syndrome (see Question **65**).
• Wernicke encephalopathy.
• Hypertrophic olivary degeneration (**52G**, axial T2).
The differential diagnosis of brainstem lesions is broad; accurate diagnosis requires consideration of patient age and specific imaging characteristics. Pontine glioma (**52E**) and metastasis (**52F**) represent the most common neoplastic lesions in children and adults, respectively. Focal areas of signal abnormality should prompt consideration of infarct or metabolic abnormality. Hypertrophic olivary degeneration (**52G**) is hypertrophy and T2 hyperintensity of the inferior olivary nucleus in response to an interruption of neuronal input along the triangle of Guillain–Mollaret, which runs from the dentate nucleus in the cerebellum via the red nucleus to the inferior olivary nucleus.

Pathology and clinical correlation CM is a benign vascular hamartoma consisting of immature blood vessels with intralesional haemorrhages and lack of neural tissue. Within CM, 75% occur as a solitary, sporadic lesion and 25% as multiple, familial lesions with earlier presentation and higher risk of bleeding than the sporadic form. CMs might occur throughout the central nervous system, although the brain, especially the brainstem, is much more often affected than the spinal cord. CMs show a very variable prognosis, because lesions might regress, enlarge, or develop *de novo*. The typical clinical presentation is a 40–60-year-old patient with seizures after bleeding.

TEACHING PEARLS (CASE 52)

> *Think of CM in middle-aged patients with spontaneous intracranial haemorrhage.*
> *CM is a round nonenhancing haemorrhagic mass (best seen in T2*GRE) with complete hemosiderin rim on T2.*
> *It is the most common angiographically occult vascular malformation.*
> *CM is most commonly located in brainstem or cerebral hemispheres.*
> *Gradient echo images are useful to identify additional lesions.*

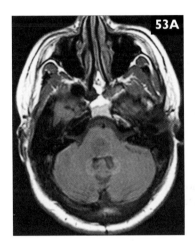
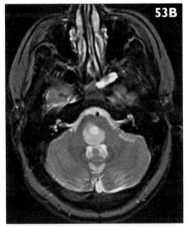

53 An adult presents with right facial droop. The following images are obtained (**53A–C**).

i. Is brainstem biopsy usually performed to confirm diagnosis?

ii. Define the anatomic boundaries of the brainstem.

iii. Name the age range most commonly affected by primary tumours of the brainstem.

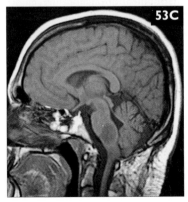

53 **DIAGNOSIS** Focal pontine brainstem glioma.

IMAGING FINDINGS There is a well-circumscribed mass within the inferior pons near the midline showing T1 hypointensity (**53A, C**) and T2 hyperintensity (**53B**). The mass is primarily solid but has a smaller cystic component anteriorly. No enhancement is observed. No other lesions are identified.

DIFFERENTIAL DIAGNOSIS Nonenhancing lesions of the brainstem are rare. Brainstem gliomas (BGs) should always be considered. Conceivably, a demyelinating disease or rhomboencephalitis could have a similar appearance but additional regions of abnormality would be expected. Correlation with clinical presentation is necessary, but the diagnosis of BG is often made by imaging alone as a biopsy carries a high risk of resultant neurological deficit (i).

PATHOLOGY AND CLINICAL CORRELATION The brainstem is generally defined as that part of the brain extending from the midbrain to the cervical junction (ii). BGs are any glial tumours primarily involving a portion of the anatomic brainstem. Lesions are generally bright on T2- and dark on T1-weighted imaging. Contrast enhancement is variable. Though all are glial in origin, tumour position and diffuse or focal pattern make them a heterogeneous group in terms of prognosis and treatment. These tumours can affect any age group but are most common in the paediatric population (iii). They show a primary peak in the latter half of the first decade and a second smaller peak in the fourth decade.

The most common form of BG is the diffuse pontine form. Unfortunately, this form also shows the worst prognosis with survival similar to that of adult supratentorial glioblastoma multiforme. Surgery is usually not feasible as there is diffuse involvement throughout the majority of the pons. Radiation therapy, with or without chemotherapy, is usually administered. Less common forms of BG are more likely to be low-grade lesions and are separated into several groups including: tectal gliomas, focal pontine gliomas (as in this case), dorsal exophytic tumours, and cervico-medullary lesions. In these less aggressive subtypes, surgery is sometimes beneficial and survival rates are considerably improved. The heterogeneous nature of the lesions makes absolute survival numbers difficult to quote with true confidence.

TEACHING PEARLS
➤ *BGs are most commonly diffuse and infiltrative.*
➤ *Focal BGs carry a better prognosis.*
➤ *Imaging findings along with clinical presentation is often used for diagnosis, with biopsies reserved for only the most confusing cases.*

REFERENCES (CASE 53)

Chamberlain MC (1999). Adult brainstem gliomas (Correspondence). *Neurology* 53(2):437–8.

Landolfi JC, Thaler HT, DeAngelis LM (1998). Adult brainstem gliomas. *Neurology* 51(4):1136–9.

Walker DA, Punt JAG, Sokal M (1999). Clinical management of brainstem glioma. *Arch Dis Child* 80:558–564.

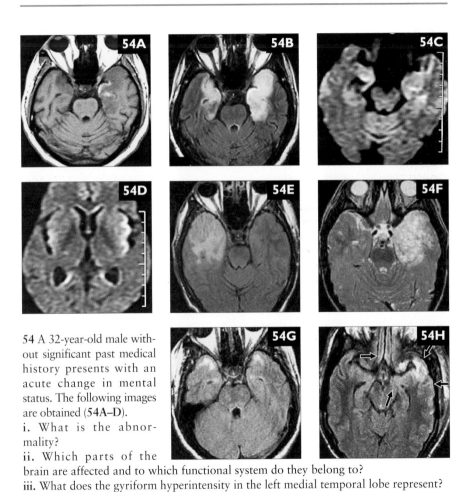

54 A 32-year-old male without significant past medical history presents with an acute change in mental status. The following images are obtained (54A–D).

i. What is the abnormality?

ii. Which parts of the brain are affected and to which functional system do they belong to?

iii. What does the gyriform hyperintensity in the left medial temporal lobe represent?

DIFFERENTIAL DIAGNOSIS Images 54E–H.

54 Diagnosis Herpes simplex encephalitis (HSE).

Imaging findings Images **54A, B** (axial T1, axial FLAIR) demonstrate bilateral but asymmetric (left greater than right) T2 hyperintense lesions (**i**) of the limbic system including the medial temporal lobes and the insulae (**ii**). These lesions are DWI bright (**54C, D**). Gyriform cortical haemorrhage is shown on the T1 sequence in the left medial temporal lobe consistent with subacute haemorrhage (**iii**).

Differential diagnosis The differential diagnosis of a temporal lobe lesion includes:
1. Considerations for bilateral temporal lobe involvement:
- HSE (**54A–D**).
- Limbic encephalitis.
- Lymphoma (see Question **69**).
2. Additional considerations if unilateral temporal lobe involvement:
- Ischaemia (posterior cerebral artery infarction).
- Ischaemia (Vein of Labbe infarct).
- Ischaemia (CADASIL) (**54G**, axial FLAIR).
- Status epilepticus.
- Glioma (e.g. glioblastoma multiforme, GBM) (**54E**, axial FLAIR).
- Dysembryoblastic neuroepithelial tumour (DNET) (**54F**, axial T2).
- Contusion (**54H**, axial FLAIR).

It is crucial to consider the diagnosis of HSE when presented with signal abnormalities corresponding to the limbic system, including the medial temporal lobes. Other differential possibilities include ischaemia (arterial, venous, or small vessel infarcts), neoplasm (GBM, lymphoma, or DNET), or contusion in the setting of trauma. A mimic of HSE is limbic encephalitis, a paraneoplastic disorder.

Pathology and clinical correlation HSE is a brain parenchyma infection that involves the limbic system and is caused by herpes simplex virus type 1 (HSV-1). Common locations include the medial temporal lobe, insula, subfrontal area, fornix, and cingulate gyrus. Late features are gyriform enhancement and subacute haemorrhage. HSE typically appears in young adults with an acute onset of seizures, fever, and headache. Even if intravenous acyclovir therapy is started immediately after diagnosis, approximately 50% of patients will suffer neurological disabilities including memory loss, hearing loss, epilepsy, and personality changes. HSE is the most common cause of fatal encephalitis, with a mortality of approximately 60%.

TEACHING PEARLS

➤ *HSE occurs with bilateral but asymmetric T2/FLAIR hyperintense lesions affecting the limbic system with restricted diffusion. Remember that while the temporal lobe is most commonly affected, any part of the limbic system can be abnormal.*

➤ *Late features (1 week after initial symptoms) include gyriform enhancement and subacute haemorrhage.*

➤ *Acute onset of symptoms and bilaterality are helpful to differentiate HSV encephalitis from other aetiologies.*

➤ *HSE can occur at any age, but the highest incidence is in adolescents and young adults.*

REFERENCES

Koeller KK, Smirniotopoulos JG, Jones RV (1997). Primary central nervous system lymphoma: radiologic-pathologic correlation. *Radiographics* 17(6):1497–526.

Kuker W, *et al.* (2004). Diffusion-weighted MRI in herpes simplex encephalitis. *Neuroradiology* 46:122–5.

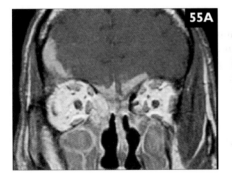 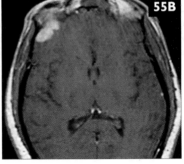

55 A 37-year-old West African female presents with headaches and fatigue. The following images (**55A, B**) are obtained.

i. What sequences are shown?

ii. What is the pattern of enhancement seen? What are the differential possibilities?

55 **Diagnosis** Neurosarcoidosis.

Imaging findings Coronal and axial T1-weighted post-gadolinium images (**55A, B**) (**i**) show enhancing dural masses along the floor of the anterior cranial fosssa. Extensive sinus disease is also noted, likely unrelated to the dural masses (**ii**).

Differential diagnosis Common differential possibilities for thick, nodular, dural based enhancement include meningioma (typically more uniform than nodular, with a dural tail), dural metastases, lymphoma/sarcoidosis (although lymphoma is more common, neurosarcoid can have a similar imaging presentation, and these two should usually be considered together), plasmacytoma and, less commonly, tuberculosis, fungal infection, or Wegeners granulomatosis (**ii**). CSF hypotension manifests as diffuse, uniform, dural enhancement and hence should not be considered here.

Pathology and clinical correlation Neurosarcoid is a multisystem inflammatory disease of unknown aetiology characterized by noncaseating epitheloid-cell granulomas. The lesions of neurosarcoid are most commonly dural or leptomeningeal, with a particular predilection for the basal cisterns (optic chiasm, hypothalamus, infundibulum, and cranial nerves). Parenchymal lesions are less common but can involve the hypothalamus. Another common presentation is multiple periventricular foci of T2 hyperintensity that can be associated with a small vessel vasculitis. Patients most commonly present with a cranial nerve palsy. The CNS is involved in 5–27% of patients with sarcoidosis, of whom 50% are asymptomatic. Corticosteroids can be used to alleviate symptoms. Enlarged hilar and mediastinal lymph nodes on chest radiographs might help to confirm the diagnosis.

Teaching pearls
> Like lymphoma, neurosarcoid is a 'great mimicker' in neuroradiology.
> It has many manifestations in the CNS: dural masses, leptomeningeal enhancement, parenchymal lesions, hypothalamus/infundibulum lesions, cranial nerves.
> Consider a chest CT to evaluate for pulmonary manifestations of sarcoid if an abnormality involves the parenchyma, meninges, and bone.
> Neurosarcoidosis is associated with small vessel vasculitis.
> It presents most commonly with cranial nerve palsy (especially facial nerve) due to coating of cranial nerves in the basilar cisterns.
> It typically occurs in young to middle-aged adults.

Reference
Hayes WS, *et al.* (1986). MR and CT evaluation of intracranial sarcoidosis. *AJR* **149**: 1043–9.

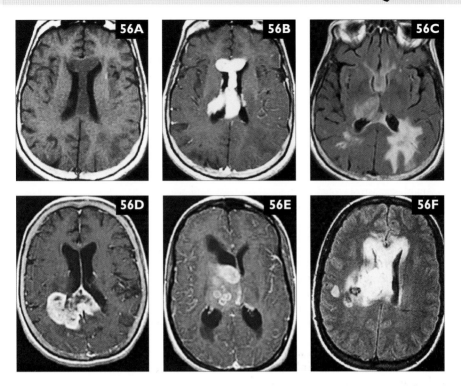

56 A 41-year-old male presents with AIDS and increasing headache, and the following images are obtained (**56A–C**).
i. What are the signal characteristics of the lesion?
ii. Where is the lesion located?
iii. What is the differential diagnosis?

DIFFERENTIAL DIAGNOSIS Images 56D–F.

56: Answer

56 Diagnosis Primary CNS lymphoma (PCNSL).

Imaging findings Images 56A–C (axial T1, axial contrast-enhanced T1, and axial FLAIR, respectively) demonstrate an intensely enhancing signal that crosses the corpus callosum and extends along the subependymal surface of the lateral ventricles bilaterally (**i, ii**).

Differential diagnosis The differential diagnosis (**iii**) of lesions that cross the corpus callosum includes:
- Lymphoma (56A–D, axial contrast-enhanced T1).
- Glioblastoma multiforme (GBM) (see Question 60).
- Anaplastic astrocytoma (56E, axial contrast-enhanced T1).
- Multiple sclerosis/demyelination.
- Shear injury (trauma).
- Rare: Marchiafava–Bignami.

The differential diagnosis of lesions that involve the septum pellucidum is central neurocytoma (56F, axial FLAIR). The differential diagnosis of lesions that cross the corpus callosum is a classic in neuroradiology that can be extremely useful in practice. Differentiating these processes may require correlation with the clinical history and symptoms. Image 56D shows heterogeneous, peripherally-enhancing lymphoma typical of an immunocompromised patient involving the right periatrial white matter and crossing the splenium of the corpus callosum. The anaplastic astrocytoma in 56E crosses the corpus callousm and shows focal round areas of enhancement. Neurocytoma is rarely malignant and might be indistinguishable from lymphoma as in 56F.

Pathology and clinical correlation PCNSL accounts for about 5% of all primary brain tumours, with rising incidence due to continuing increase of HIV infection. PCNSL is an AIDS defining condition with an incidence of about 4% in these patients. Dramatic response to steroids and radiation therapy in PCNSL does not improve the dismal prognosis of patients with this lesion. Steroid therapy has a dramatic effect on imaging and biopsy results.

Teaching pearls
➢ *Periventricular, subependymal, and corpus callosum involvement is typical of PCNSL.*
➢ *The most common lesions that cross the corpus callosum include: lymphoma, GBM, demyelination, shear injury.*
➢ *Multifocal and multicompartmental distribution is characteristic for lymphoma.*
➢ *PCNSL is hyperdense on NECT, due to dense cellularity, T2 hypointense, T1 hypointense, and strongly enhancing mass on MR.*
➢ *Like neurosarcoid, lymphoma is a 'great mimicker', with many manifestations in the CNS.*

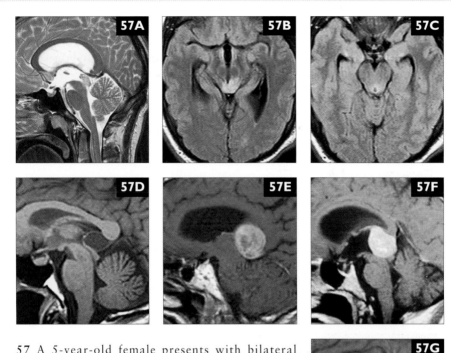

57 A 5-year-old female presents with bilateral papilloedema, headache, and vomiting. The following images are obtained (57A–C).
i. Which structures are involved?
ii. Which complication could be expected with a lesion in this location (not obviously present in this case)?
iii. How does location relate to prognosis and clinical outcome?

DIFFERENTIAL DIAGNOSIS Images 57D–G.

57 DIAGNOSIS Tectal glioma.

IMAGING FINDINGS Images 57A–C (sagittal T2, axial FLAIR, axial FLAIR, respectively) demonstrate a T2/FLAIR hyperintense lesion involving the tectum and the periaqueductal grey of the midbrain (i). The tumour can cause obstructive hydrocephalus (ii) by obstructing the aqueduct with enlargement of the 3rd ventricle and the body of the lateral ventricle.

DIFFERENTIAL DIAGNOSIS The differential diagnosis of a pineal region mass includes:
- Pineal cyst (57D, sagittal T1).
- Pineocytoma (see Question 67).
- Pineoblastoma.
- Tectal glioma (57A–C).
- Meningioma (57E; sagittal contrast-enhanced T1).
- Metastasis (57F; sagittal contrast-enhanced T1).
- Germ cell tumour.
- Corpus callosum lipoma (57G, sagittal T1).
- See also differential diagnosis for pineal region mass in Question 18.

Image 57D shows a homogenous fluid filled pineal cyst clearly distinct from the tectum. Image 57E demonstrates an enhancing pineal region meningioma, which usually arise from the tentorium or falx cerebelli. The intensely enhancing melanoma in 57F is almost indistinguishable from a meningioma. The corpus callosum lipoma shown in 57G is characterized by intrinsic T1 hyperintensity; lipomas can be associated with other developmental abnormalities of the brain.

PATHOLOGY AND CLINICAL CORRELATION Tectal gliomas are usually low-grade astrocytomas that enlarge the tectum and may completely obliterate the aqueduct of Sylvius, causing hydrocephalus. In this case, patients typically present with neurological symptoms resulting from increased intracranial pressure. Unlike other brainstem gliomas, tectal gliomas have a favourable prognosis (iii). Usually they show low-grade histology. Although they are not amenable to resection, shunting is all that is needed to allow long-term survival in many cases.

TEACHING PEARLS
➤ *Consider tectal glioma in a young child presenting with hydrocephalus.*
➤ *T2/FLAIR is hyperintense, usually minimally or nonenhancing lesion originating from the quadrigeminal plate.*
➤ *Tectal glioma has a good prognosis compared to other gliomas.*
➤ *Shunting of hydrocephalus is the primary treatment.*
➤ *Mean patient age is 6 years.*

REFERENCE
Osborn AG, *et al.* (2004). *Brain.* Amirsys, Salt Lake City, Chapter I-6, pp. 88–91.

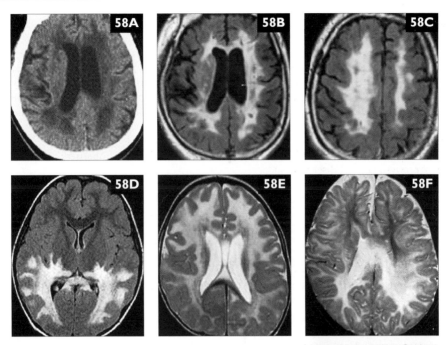

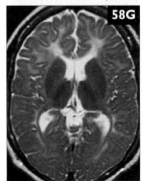

58 A 33-year-old female with recurrent episodes of transient ischaemic attacks (TIAs) presents, and the following images are obtained (**58A–C**).
i. Which part of the brain is affected?
ii. How was this abnormality acquired by the patient?
iii. What other disorders could have a similar appearance?

DIFFERENTIAL DIAGNOSIS Images 58D–G.

58: Answer

58 Diagnosis Cerebral autosomal dominant arteriopathy with subcortical infarct and leukoencephalopathy (CADASIL).

Imaging findings Images 58A–C (axial unenhanced CT and two FLAIR images, respectively) demonstrate a confluent bilateral asymmetric leukoencephalopathy involving the periventricular white matter (WM), the centrum semiovale, and the subcortical U-fibres (i). The lesion is hypodense on unenhanced CT and hyperintense on the FLAIR sequence.

Differential diagnosis The differential diagnosis (iii) of an inherited confluent periventricular WM disease includes:
- Metachromatic leukodystrophy (MLD) (see Question 61).
- X-linked adrenoleukodystrophy (X-ALD) (58D, axial FLAIR).
- CADASIL (58A–C).
- Alexander disease (58E, axial T2).
- Canavan disease (58F, axial T2).
- Pelizaeus–Merzbacher disease (58G, axial T2).

Other confluent WM processes include:
- Progressive multifocal leukoencephalopathy (PML).
- Post-radiation change.

X-ALD (58D) is an inherited disorder of peroxisome metabolism with enhancing demyelination of the peritrigonal WM and the splenium, typically diagnosed in preteen males. Alexander disease (58E) is a leukoencephalopathy characterized by diffuse symmetrical bifrontal WM disease in macrocephalic infants. Canavan disease (58F) is a progressive autosomal recessive leukodystrophy with diffuse confluent demyelination and early U-fibre involvement; MRS shows a marked spike of n-acetyl aspartate. Pelizaeus–Merzbacher disease (58G) is a X-linked leukodystrophy with diffuse brain atrophy, bilateral symmetric WM T2 hyperintensities, and T2 hypointensities in the thalami and lentiform nuclei.

Pathology and clinical correlation CADASIL is a hereditary small-vessel disease due to mutation of the notch 3 gene on chromosome 19, which causes subcortical lacunar infarcts and leukoencephalopathy in young adults (ii). The most common locations are the frontal lobe, temporal lobe, periventricular WM, and centrum semiovale. Patients typically develop migraine in the 3rd–4th decades, transient ischaemic attacks and strokes in 4th–5th decades, and dementia in the 6th–7th decades.

Teaching pearls
> *Consider CADASIL in young patients with recurrent ischaemic attacks and leukoencephalopathy.*
> *Angiography is normal in CADASIL.*
> *Anterior temporal lobe and external capsule involvement might help differentiate CADASIL from other leukoencephalopathies.*

REFERENCES (CASE 58)
Oberstein L, *et al.* (2003). Incipient CADASIL. *Arch Neurol* **60**:707–12.
Osborn AG, *et al.* (2004). *Brain.* Amirsys, Salt Lake City, Chapter I-9, pp. 28–57.

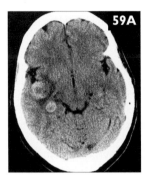

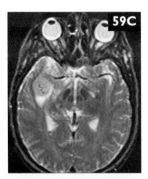

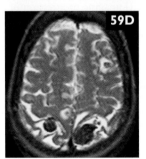

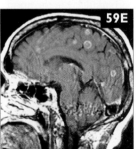

59 A patient presents with decreased level of cons-ciousness. The following images are obtained (**59A–E**).

i. What are several causes of multiple non-neoplastic cerebral intraparenchymal haemorrhage?

ii. What primary tumours classically produce haem-orrhagic metastases?

iii. Describe the normal MRI imaging progression of blood product?

59 DIAGNOSIS Haemorrhagic metastases.

IMAGING FINDINGS Multiple intraparenchymal hyperdensities are seen on CT (**59A, B**) suggestive of haemorrhage. T2-weighted MRI shows variable signal within the corresponding lesions indicating blood products of varying age (**59C, D**). Sagittal postcontrast T1 image reveals multiple enhancing masses highly suggestive of metastatic disease (**59E**).

DIFFERENTIAL DIAGNOSIS The differential for multiple cerebral haemorrhagic lesions is trauma, haemorrhagic metastases, multiple familial cavernous malformations, amyloid angiopathy, and hypertensive microhaemorrhages (**i**).

PATHOLOGY AND CLINICAL CORRELATION Haemorrhagic metastases are encountered with a number of primary neoplasms including renal cell carcinoma, melanoma, colon carcinoma, testicular tumours, and others (**ii**). When evaluating multiple intracranial intraparenchymal haemorrhages it important to consider haemorrhagic metastases. Clinical history is often very helpful. Several imaging signs suggest this diagnosis as well. First, enhancing masses either clearly related to the haemorrhages or distinct from them (as in this case) usually make the diagnosis straightforward. However, enhancement can occasionally be difficult to differentiate from subacute intrinsic T1 hyperintensity. Second, delay in the normal MRI imaging progression of blood product can be a clue to haemorrhagic neoplasm and is felt to be due to differing oxygen tensions relative to normal brain. The usual non-neoplastic MRI progression is as follows (**iii**):

Stage	T1	T2
Hyperacute	isointense	iso/bright
Acute	isointense	dark
Subacute (early)	bright	dark
Subacute (late)	bright	bright
Chronic	iso/dark	dark

TEACHING PEARLS
- *Contrast enhancement related to multiple intraparenchymal haemorrhages is highly suggestive of haemorrhagic metastases.*
- *Delay in the usual MRI progression of blood product can be seen with intratumoural haemorrhage due to differing oxygen tension as compared to normal brain.*

REFERENCES
Bradley WG Jr (1993). MR appearance of haemorrhage in the brain. *Radiology* 189(1):15–26.
Destian S, *et al.* (1989). MR imaging of haemorrhagic intracranial neoplasms. *AJR* 152(1):137–44.

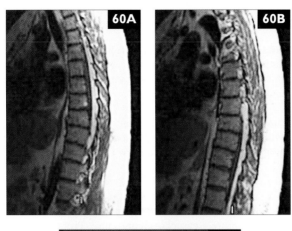

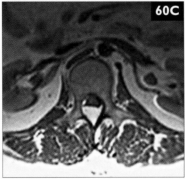

60 A 32-year-old man presents with difficulty walking and the following images are obtained (**60A–C**).
i. What substance is compressing the thecal sac?
ii. How can it be treated?

60 **DIAGNOSIS**   Epidural lipomatosis.

IMAGING FINDINGS   Sagittal and axial T1-weighted images show a diffuse T1 hyperintense mass within the posterior epidural space. It shows the same signal as fat (i) (compare with subcutaneous fat). The axial image shows that it exerts mass effect on the thecal sac, which is flattened posteriorly.

DIFFERENTIAL DIAGNOSIS   The main differential diagnosis of an epidural mass showing pre-contrast T1 hyperintensity is an epidural haematoma. Encapsulated spinal lipomas should also be distinguished from lipomatosis.

PATHOLOGY AND CLINICAL CORRELATION   Epidural lipomatosis is a rare condition, more commonly seen in males. Predisposing factors include obesity and steroid administration. Symptoms develop slowly and likely reflect direct mechanical compression as well as indirect vascular compromise. Progressive myelopathy is the most common finding, as the thoracic region is most commonly involved. Treatment is usually by weight loss or steroid reduction, but occasionally surgery is required (ii).

TEACHING PEARLS
➤ *An epidural lipoma can be distinguished from a hematoma by fat saturated images.*
➤ *Epidural adipose tissue that has a thickness greater than 7 mm has been suggested as a diagnostic criterion for epidural lipomatosis.*

REFERENCE
Robertson SC, *et al.* (1997) Idiopathic spinal epidural lipomatosis. *Neurosurgery* **41**:68–75.

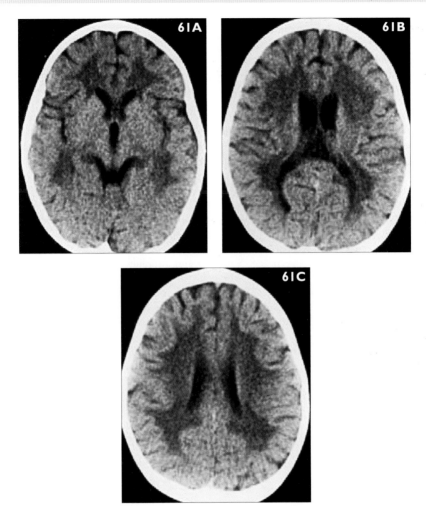

61 A 9-year-old male presents with poor performance in school and motor difficulty.
i. Where is the abnormality on these axial images CT images (61A–C)?
ii. What is the underlying abnormality?

61 DIAGNOSIS Metachromatic leukodystrophy (MLD).

IMAGING FINDINGS Images 61A–C show confluent periventricular white matter hypodensity in a typical 'butterfly' pattern, with relative sparing of the subcortical U-fibres (i).

DIFFERENTIAL DIAGNOSIS The key finding is a confluent white matter abnormality in a paediatric male. Differential possibilities in this cohort include primarily metabolic abnormalities, such as MLD, X-linked adrenoleukodysyrophy, CADASIL, Alexander disease, Canavan disease, and Pelizaeus–Merzbacker disease. There is no history of radiation exposure to explain the white matter findings.

PATHOLOGY AND CLINICAL CORRELATION MLD is the most common hereditary leukodystrophy, caused by insufficient activity of the enzyme arylsulfatase A (ii). The most common form of MLD is the late infantile form with manifestation between 1 and 2 years, presenting with ataxia and hypotonia. Lifespan is typically 8–10 years. A Juvenile form appears between ages 5 and 10 and an adult form can mimic MS and present in the 3rd and 4th decades. MR can demonstrate restricted diffusion at the frontier of active demyelination. Differentiation is aided by the characteristic pattern of involvement, lack of enhancement (a feature of MLD shared by progressive multifocal leukoencephalopathy [PML], although the latter occurs only in immunocompromised patients), and elevated choline in the affected white matter on MR spectroscopy. Head size is also an important differentiating feature; it is typically elevated with Canavan's and Alexander's diseases, but age appropriate with MLD.

TEACHING PEARLS
➤ *MLD is the most common hereditary leukodystrophy.*
➤ *There is characteristic 'butterfly pattern' of cerebral hemispheric WM with early sparing of subcortical U-fibres.*
➤ *Lack of enhancement is seen.*
➤ *There are late infantile, juvenile, and adult forms.*

REFERENCES
Faerber EN, Melvin J, Smergel EM (1999). MRI appearance of metachromatic leukodystrophy. *Pediatr Radiol* **29**(9):669–72.
Osborn AG, *et al.* (2004). *Brain*, Amirsys, Salt Lake City, Chapter I-9, pp. 28–57.

62 A patient presents with left-sided sensorineural hearing loss, and the following images are obtained (62A, B).

i. Name the two components of the eighth cranial nerve (CN VIII).

ii. Describe the anatomic relationship of CN VII to CN VIII within the internal auditory canal.

iii. What is the classic differential diagnosis for cerebellopontine angle masses?

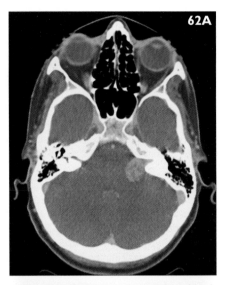

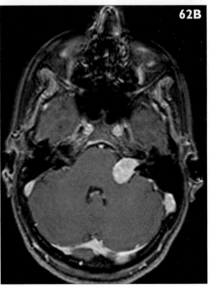

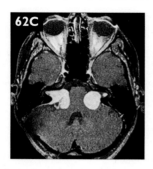
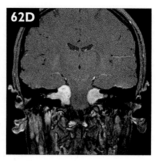

62 DIAGNOSIS Acoustic schwannoma.

IMAGING FINDINGS Image **62A** is a contrast-enhanced CT scan showing a focal mass within the left cerebellopontine angle (CPA) and internal auditory canal (IAC). The window and level settings are such that osseous expansion of the proximal IAC is readily apparent. This mass is confirmed by MRI (**62B**) which shows it to be a single avidly enhancing lesion causing mass effect on the adjacent middle cerebellar peduncle.

The companion case (**62C, D**) demonstrates bilateral homogeneously enhancing CPA/IAC masses on postcontrast T1 axial (**62C**) and coronal (**62D**) images.

DIFFERENTIAL DIAGNOSIS The classic radiographic differential diagnosis for enhancing CPA mass lesions is acoustic schwannoma (by far the most common) and meningioma, followed by less common lesions including ependymoma (iii). Extension of the tumour into the IAC with resultant osseous remodelling strongly favours acoustic schwannoma.

PATHOLOGY AND CLINICAL CORRELATION CN VIII has two main components: the vestibular and cochlear portions (i). The VIIth and VIIIth cranial nerves travel together within the IAC, with the VIIth nerve superior to the cochlear portion and anterior to the two subdivisions of the vestibular portion (ii). It is the vestibular portion that is most commonly affected by acoustic schwannomas, providing the more accurate synonym vestibular schwannoma. 'Acoustic neuroma' is a misnomer and should not be used.

These benign slow-growing tumours arise from Schwann cells of the nerve sheath and most often present in adults with unilateral sensorineural hearing loss. The lesions can be quite small at presentation, so careful evaluation of the CPA and IAC is required. Treatment is variable with radiation therapy (gamma knife), surgery, and watchful waiting all accepted options.

By definition, patients with bilateral acoustic schwannomas have neurofibromatosis type 2 (NF2). NF2 is an autosomal dominant disorder accounting for approximately 3% of all cases of neurofibromatosis. It is, therefore, much less common than NF1. The term MISME (multiple inherited schwannomas, meningiomas, and ependymomas) has become widely used as a mneumonic to remember this disease.

62: Answer

TEACHING PEARLS
➤ *Acoustic schwannoma is by far the most common CPA mass.*
➤ *Acoustic schwannomas are slow-growing benign tumours arising from the nerve sheath of the vestibular portion of CN VIII.*
➤ *Bilateral acoustic schwannomas are neurofibromatosis Type 2 by definition.*

REFERENCES
Khurana VG, *et al.* (2003).Evolution of a cochlear schwannoma on clinical and neuroimaging studies. *J Neurosurg* **99**(4):779–82.
Raut VV, *et al.* (2004). Conservative management of vestibular schwannomas: second review of a prospective longitudinal study. *Clin Otolaryngol Allied Sci* **29**(5):505–14.
Rodriguez D, Poussaint TY (2004). Neuroimaging findings in neurofibromatosis type 1 and 2. *Neuroimag Clin N Am* **14**:149–70.

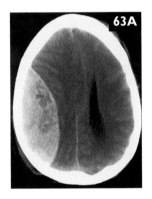 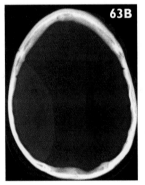 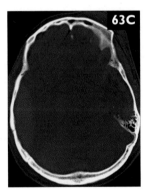

63 A patient presents after a multiple vehicle accident, with initial brief loss of consciousness, but is now alert and oriented. The following images are obtained (63A–C).
i. Haemorrhage into which extra-axial space produces this lentiform appearance?
ii. Are arteries or veins more commonly injured with this form of haemorrhage?
iii. Which type of extra-axial haemorrhage is limited by the falx cerebri?

63 DIAGNOSIS Epidural haematoma (EDH).

IMAGING FINDINGS Image **63A** shows a classic biconvex, lentiform, extra-axial, hyperdense, epidural haematoma on the right (**i**). Blood product extends from the sagittal suture anteriorly to the lambdoid suture posteriorly (**63B**) and there is a nondisplaced linear skull fracture visible adjacent to the central portion of the haematoma (**63C**).

DIFFERENTIAL DIAGNOSIS Differential considerations include subdural (SDH) and intraparenchymal (IPH) haematomas. When large extra-axial haematomas are encountered, as in this case, there is little difficulty placing the haematoma in the correct space. Smaller haematomas can occasionally be difficult to define. EDHs are differentiated from SDHs primarily by shape and location. EDHs are convex and can cross the falx but not suture lines. SDHs, on the other hand, classically show crescentic shape and can cross suture lines but not the falx (**iii**). IPHs, as the name implies, are entirely intraparenchymal.

PATHOLOGY AND CLINICAL CORRELATION EDHs are found in 1–4% of patients imaged for craniocerebral trauma. A classic 'lucid interval' between the trauma and neurological deterioration is often described in the literature but is seen in only about half of patients with EDH. Delayed development or enlargement is seen in up to 30% of EDHs and usually occurs within the first 48 hours following trauma. EDHs are associated with skull fractures (most commonly lacerating the middle meningeal artery) in 85–95% of cases (**ii**). Occasionally, the fracture is best demonstrated on the CT scout image. Overall mortality is approximately 5% and standard treatment is by surgical evacuation.

TEACHING PEARLS
➤ *EDHs are convex extra-axial haematomas that do not cross suture margins.*
➤ *They are most often associated with linear skull fractures that lacerate the middle meningeal artery.*
➤ *Standard treatment is by emergent surgical evacuation.*
➤ *A history of a 'lucid interval' is present in only half of patients with EDHs.*

REFERENCES
Osborn A (1994). *Diagnostic Neuroradiology*. Mosby, St Louis, pp. 204–5.
Sullivan TP, Jarvik JG, Cohen WA (1999). Follow-up of conservatively managed epidural haematomas: implications for timing of repeat CT. *AJNR* **20**(1):107–13.

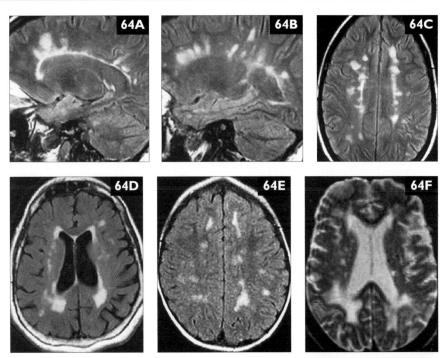

64 A 32-year-old female presents with double vision and left hand numbness, and the following images are obtained (**64A–C**).

i. Where is the hyperintense thin stripe in image **64A** localized?

ii. Which structure do the ovoid hyperintensities follow on image **64B, C**?

iii What is the specific name of these lesions mentioned in (ii)?

iv. What additional MR studies would you recommend in this disease?

DIFFERENTIAL DIAGNOSIS Images 64D–G.

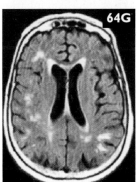

64: Answer

64 DIAGNOSIS Multiple sclerosis (MS).

IMAGING FINDINGS Image **64A** (sagittal FLAIR) demonstrates a hyperintense callososeptal striation following the corpus callosum (**i**). Image **64B** (sagittal FLAIR) shows the typical appearance of Dawson's fingers (**iii**) which are lesions aligned perpendicular to the ependymal lining of the lateral ventricles along the path of deep medullary veins (**ii**).

DIFFERENTIAL DIAGNOSIS The differential diagnosis of multifocal punctate periventricular lesions includes:
- Microangiopathy (**64D**, axial FLAIR).
- MS (**64A–C**).
- Acute disseminated encephalomyelitis (ADEM) (**64E**, axial FLAIR).
- Vasculitis (**64F**, axial T2).
- Lymphoma (**64G**, axial FLAIR).
- Lyme disease (see Question **68**).
- Sarcoidosis.
- Enlarged perivascular spaces (Virchow–Robin spaces).

Image **64D** shows periventricular white matter FLAIR hyperintensities in small-vessel disease (microangiopathy), a common finding in elderly patients. ADEM in **64E** resembles MS on imaging and might only be distinguished by a monophasic course and a history of infection or vaccination 10–14 days prior to onset of neurological symptoms. Vasculitis (**64F**), especially chronic granulomatous angiitis, might mimic MS or microangiopathic change; the diagnosis of vasculitis is confirmed by characteristic beading of vessels on angiography. Lymphoma (**64G**) should be considered in the differential diagnosis in the correct clinical setting.

PATHOLOGY AND CLINICAL CORRELATION MS is a probable autoimmune-mediated demyelination disorder in genetically susceptible individuals. The exact aetiology is still unknown at this time. MS is the leading cause of nontraumatic neurological disability in young and middle-aged adults affecting 2,500,000 people worldwide, especially Caucasians in temperate zones. 85% of MS patients suffer from a relapsing–remitting course. Common presentations include optic neuritis, weakness, numbness, tingling, and gait disturbances. Classically, the diagnosis of MS requires the presence of multiple lesions, 'separated in space and time'. The presence of enhancement is associated with active demyelination; this can be used to differentiate older plaques (without enhancement) from active lesions (with enhancement). The presence of a single lesion in the brain can be a diagnostic dilemma; screening the spine for additional lesions is a useful adjunctive study in this setting (**iv**). Other clinical exams that can be performed include auditory evoked potentials. Evaluation for possible optic neuritis may require a specifically tailored protocol that evaluates the optic nerves to best advantage.

TEACHING PEARLS (CASE 64)

➤ *Periventricular and callososeptal WM disease, with perivenular extension ('Dawson fingers') is characteristic of MS.*

➤ *T1 'holes', although potentially oedematous and reversible, tend to correlate with irreversible chronic progressive disease when cavitated.*

➤ *The proportion of T2 hyperintense lesion/T1 hypointense lesions (T1/T2 ratio) is an important parameter of chronic and persistent defect.*

➤ *Recently, the progressive forms of MS have been shown to involve not only reversible myelin damage, but also axonal transection and direct neuronal injury.*

➤ *There is transient enhancement during active demyelination.*

➤ *95% of clinically definite MS patients have positive MR.*

➤ *Mean onset age: 30 years.*

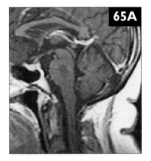
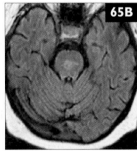
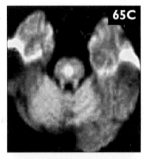

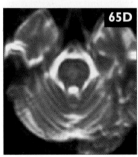

65 A homeless adult male is admitted with change in mental status and a metabolic abnormality. He develops seizures soon after admission.

i. Where are the findings on the MR images and their location (**65A–D**)?

ii. What is the differential diagnosis?

65 DIAGNOSIS Osmotic demyelination syndrome

IMAGING FINDINGS Images 65A–D (sagittal T1 postgadolinium, axial FLAIR, DWI, axial T2, respectively) show a nonenhancing region of T1 hypointensity and T2 hyperintensity in the central pons associated with restricted diffusion (i). (Note on the sagittal post-contrast images that the deep venous hyperintesity of the internal cerebral veins and straight sinus reflect gadolinium enhancement, and not T1-bright thrombus).

DIFFERENTIAL DIAGNOSIS The differential diagnosis focuses on both the clinical history and the location of the lesion in the central pons. The differential for a lesion in the brainstem in an adult includes neoplasm (metastasis, glioma), infarct, demyelination, osmotic demyelination, metablic disease, cavernous malformation, NF1, and hypertrophic olivary degeneration (ii). Paraneoplastic syndromes more commonly manifest as T2 hyperintense signal in the cerebellum or limbic structures.

PATHOLOGY AND CLINICAL CORRELATION Osmotic demyelination is classically seen in an alcoholic, hyponatraemic patient in whom rapid correction of serum sodium leads to rapid shifts in serum osmolality, resulting in extensive demyelination and gliosis. Other clinical scenarios include chronic renal failure, liver disease, DM, and SIADH. The central pons is the most common location, although supratentorial abnormalities (basal ganglia and thalamus) are seen in 50% of cases. MR is the preferred modality given its sensitivity. Clinical presentation can include seizures and altered mental status. The spectrum of prognosis ranges from complete recovery to death.

TEACHING PEARLS
➤ *The classic clinical scenario is an alcoholic, hyponatremic patient in whom rapid correction of serum sodium leads to rapid shifts in serum osmolality.*
➤ *Osmotic demyelination syndrome is preferred to the previous terminology, central pontine myelinolysis and extrapontine myelinolysis.*
➤ *Most common finding is T2 hyperintense lesions in the pons or basal ganglia.*
➤ *Lesions are T2 hyperintense with restricted diffusion. Normal signal in two rounded areas in the central pons reflects sparing of the corticospinal tracts.*
➤ *Typical clinical presentations include seizures and altered mental status.*
➤ *There is a spectrum of prognosis, from complete recovery to death.*

REFERENCES
Chua GC, *et al.* (2002). MRI findings in osmotic myelinolysis. *Clin Radiol* 57(9):800–6.
Grossman RI (2003). *Neuroradiology*, 2nd edn. Mosby, Philadelphia, pp. 355–6.

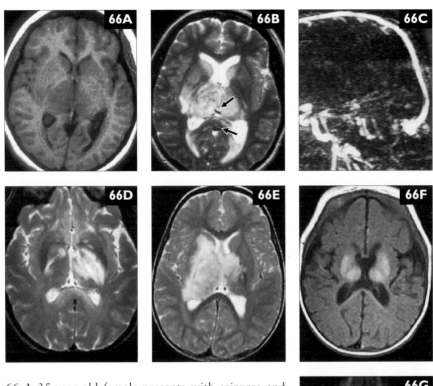

66 A 35-year-old female presents with seizures and vomiting, and the following images are obtained (66A–C).

i. Which sequences are shown?

ii. Which structures are involved?

iii. What does image 66C reveal?

iv. To what structure do the arrows in image 66B point?

DIFFERENTIAL DIAGNOSIS Images 66D–G.

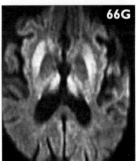

66 DIAGNOSIS Deep cerebral venous thrombosis.

IMAGING FINDINGS Images **66A–C** (axial T1, axial T2, and 2D time-of-flight [TOF] MR venography [MRV], respectively) (**i**) demonstrate a T1 hypointense and T2 hyperintense ischaemic region affecting mainly the thalami and the heads of the caudate nuclei bilaterally, right greater than left, causing mass effect with midline shift to the left side (**ii**). MRV (**66C**) reveals that there is absence of flow-related enhancement in the straight sinus, vein of Galen, and internal cerebral veins (**iii**). On the T2-weighted image (**66B**), hypointense clot in the vein of Galen (white arrow) and internal cerebral veins (black arrow) mimic normal flow voids (**iv**).

DIFFERENTIAL DIAGNOSIS The differential diagnosis of bilaterally symmetric deep nuclei lesions includes:
• Deep cerebral venous thrombosis (**66A–C**).
• Artery of Persheron infarct.
• Lymphoma (**66D**, axial T2).
• Epstein–Barr virus encephalitis.
• Japanese encephalitis.
• Eastern equine encephalitis.
• Murray valley encephalitis.
• Wernicke encephalopathy (see Question **69**).
• Bithalamic astrocytoma (**66E**, axial T2).
• Hypoxia (**66F**, axial FLAIR).
• Carbon monoxide poisoning (**66G**, axial DWI).
• Creutzfeld–Jakob disease.
• Enlarged perivascular spaces.
The differential diagnosis for bithalamic lesions includes infarct, neoplasm, infection, and metabolic disorders. Neoplasms, especially lymphoma (**66D**), with its prevalence for a multifocal and periventricular distribution, and bithalamic astrocytoma, crossing midline at the massa intermedia (**66E**), should be in the differential diagnosis of a bilateral deep nuclei lesion. Infarcts could be either venous or arterial: look for secondary signs of vascular occlusion. Metabolic disorders show typically very symmetric distribution with no mass effect: **66G** demonstrates very symmetric hyperintense signal on DWI in the deep grey nuclei, especially in the globus pallidus and in the head of the caudate nucleus bilaterally, representing carbon monoxide poisoning. In **66F**, hypoxic injury causes hyperintensity in the thalami and lentiform nuclei bilaterally.

PATHOLOGY AND CLINICAL CORRELATION Deep cerebral venous thrombosis usually affects the internal cerebral veins, vein of Galen, and straight sinus. Deep venous thrombosis can occur at any age, although elderly or debilitated patients are more likely to have spontaneous thrombosis. Most common associated symptoms are headache, nausea, vomiting, and seizure. Clincal risk factors include dehydration, pregnancy, or familial hypercoagulable states. It is important to consider the diagnosis, since the clinical symptoms are nonspecific.

TEACHING PEARLS

➤ *Always consider venous thrombosis for strokes that do not conform to arterial territory distributions.*

➤ *Always consider deep cerebral venous thrombosis in the differential of bilateral deep cerebral nuclei lesions, particularly bithalamic lesions.*

➤ *Consider lymphoma in any bilaterally symmetric neoplastic process.*

➤ *Clot in deep cerebral veins is hyperdense on NECT and can be hypointense on T2.*

➤ *2D TOF should not be interpreted without benefit of standard imaging sequences.*

➤ *Outcome is extremely variable, from asymptomatic to death.*

REFERENCES

Ding J, *et al.* (2004). Alcohol intake and cerebral abnormalities on magnetic resonance imaging in a community-based population of middle-aged adults. *Stroke* 35:16–21.

Lafitte F, *et al.* (1999). Deep cerebral vein thrombosis: imaging in eight cases. *Neuroradiology* 41:410–18.

---

67 An 18-year-old female presents with frequent headaches and visual changes.

i. What structure is involved in this sagittal T1, contrast-enhanced image (**67**)?

ii. What is the differential diagnosis for a lesion in this location?

iii. What laboratory tests may help narrow the differential diagnosis?

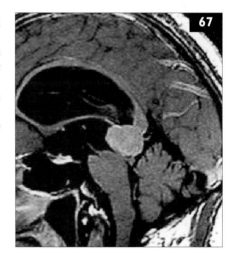

67 **DIAGNOSIS** Pineocytoma.

IMAGING FINDINGS Image 67 shows a mildly heterogeneous enhancing mass of the pineal gland (i).

DIFFERENTIAL DIAGNOSIS The differential diagnosis of a pineal region mass includes pineal cyst, pineocytoma, pineoblastoma, germ cell tumour, meningioma, metastasis, and tectal glioma. See Question 57 for a complete discussion. Gender plays an important role in ordering the differential diagnosis: 80% of pineal masses in men are germ cell tumours, whereas pineal masses in women are approximately evenly split between germ cell tumours and pineal cell tumours (pineocytoma/pineoblastoma) (ii).

PATHOLOGY AND CLINICAL CORRELATION Pineocytoma is a slow growing tumour that occurs most commonly in young adults. Symptoms are related to location, including headaches, other signs of increased intracranial pressure, and Parinaud syndrome (paralysis of upward gaze). Treatment usually involves surgical resection. Differentiation from germ cell tumours can be based on appearance (pineal cell tumours will peripherally displace pineal calcifications, whereas germ cell tumours tend to engulf pineal calcification) and serum markers (pineocytoma will result in negative tests for alpha-fetoprotein and human chorionic gonadotropin) (iii).

TEACHING PEARLS
➤ *Gender plays an important role in ordering the differential diagnosis in pineal masses, as discussed above.*
➤ *Pineocytomas are round, well-circumscribed T2 hyperintense masses with solid or peripheral enhancement.*

REFERENCES
Nakamura M, *et al.* (2000). Neuroradiological characteristic of pineocytoma and pineoblastoma. *Neuroradiology* 42(7):509–14.
Osborn AG, *et al.* (2004). *Brain.* Amirsys, Salt Lake City, Chapter I-6, pp. 88–91.

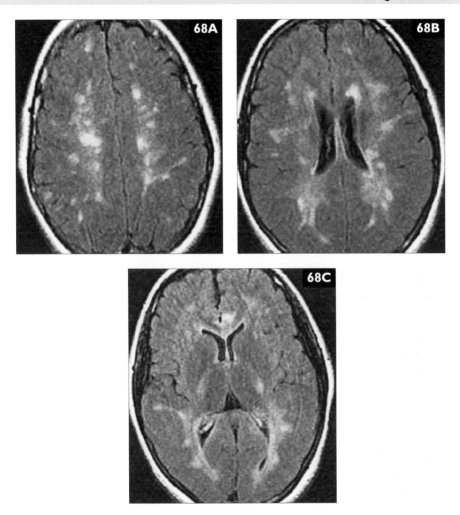

68 A 28-year-old female presents with subacute onset of vague neurological complaints and joint pain, beginning after outdoor camping in a New England wooded area.
i. What is the distribution of this abnormality (68A–C)?
ii. How is this entity transmitted?

68 **DIAGNOSIS** Lyme disease.

IMAGING FINDINGS Images 68A–C show bilateral ovoid FLAIR hyperintensities in the centrum semiovale, becoming confluent inferiorly in the periventricular white matter and internal capsule (i).

DIFFERENTIAL DIAGNOSIS The differential hinges on the periventricular distribution of the T2 hyperintense parenchymal signal abnormality. Major considerations include hypertensive microangiopathy, MS, acute disseminated encepahlomyelitis (ADEM), vasculitis, lymphoma, and Lyme disease. Narrowing the differential depends on patient demographics and clinical history.

PATHOLOGY AND CLINICAL CORRELATION Lyme disease is an inflammatory disorder triggered by a spirochaetal infection (*Borrelia burgdorferi*) transmitted by the deer tick (ii). Lyme should always be considered in the initial workup of MS, as both its diagnosis and treatment are straightforward, inexpensive, and reliable. Numerous T2 hyperintense lesions of the periventricular white matter, spinal cord, and cranial nerves (particularly CN7) are typical when there is CNS involvement (neuroborreliosis). Symptoms depend on the stage of disease, ranging from fevers, myalgias, headaches, and a petechial rash early in the disease, erythema migrans, arthralgias, and myalgias in early disseminated disease, and more severe arthritis, carditis, and CNS lesions in late disseminated disease. Early diagnosis is key as the infection responds to antibiotics if treated early (doxycycline, amoxicillin, and ceftin are the three oral antibiotics most highly recommended).

TEACHING PEARLS
➢ Always *rule out Lyme disease in patients with findings suspicious for MS, because of easy, accurate, inexpensive diagnosis and treatment.*
➢ *Lesions simulate MS in patients with skin rash and influenza-like illness.*
➢ *Location: periventricular white matter, facial nerve, cauda equina, leptomeninges.*

REFERENCE
Agosta F, *et al.* (2006). MR imaging asssesment of brain and cervical cord damage in patients with neuroborreliosis. *AJNR* **27**: 892–4.

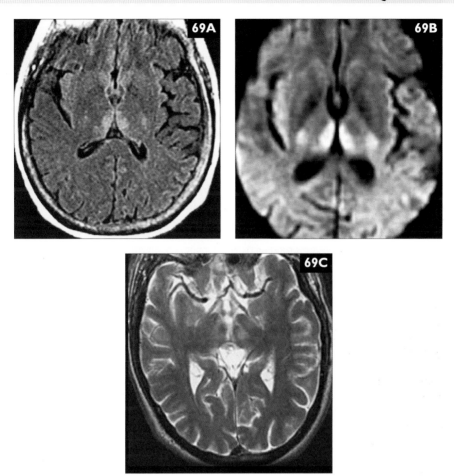

69 A 60-year-old male presents with long-standing progressive ataxia and confusion.
i. Which sequences are shown (69A–C)?
ii. What structures are involved? What is the differential diagnosis?

69 DIAGNOSIS Wernicke encephalopathy.

IMAGING FINDINGS Images 69A–C (axial FLAIR, DWI, and axial T2, respectively [i]) demonstrate FLAIR/T2 hyperintense lesions in the dorsal medial thalamic nuclei with associated restricted diffusion (ii). (ADC maps, not shown, confirm that the elevated signal on DWI correspond to restricted diffusion rather than T2 shine-through effects.)

DIFFERENTIAL DIAGNOSIS A key differential in this case is that of bilaterally symmetrical deep nuclei lesions (ii).
- Vascular (deep cerebral venous thrombosis, artery of Persheron infarct).
- Neoplastic (lymphoma [typically enhances], astrocytomas [may or may not enhance]).
- Infectious (EBV encephalitis, Japanese encephalitis, eastern equine encephalitis, Murray Valley encephalitis, Creutzfeld–Jakob disease).
- Metabolic (Wernicke's encephalopathy, CO poisoning, hypoxia).

PATHOLOGY AND CLINICAL CORRELATION Wernicke's encephalopathy results from thiamine deficiency, leading to cell damage. Although 50% of patients are alcoholic, a similar percentage of patients develop similar thiamine deficiency due to other causes, including end-stage malignancy and bone marrow transplant. Major imaging manifestations include hyperintensity in both medial thalami, the hypothalamus, and the periaqueductal grey matter. Atrophy of mamillary bodies is another important imaging finding.

TEACHING PEARLS
➤ *Classic clinical triad: ataxia, oculomotor abnormalities, confusion.*
➤ *Caused by thiamine deficiency which results in glutamate accumulation and cell damage; acute treatment is with thiamine administration (must be given prior to i.v. glucose which may precipitate an acute Wernicke's crisis).*
➤ *Imaging findings include T2 hyperintensity in both medial thalami, the hypothalamus, and the periaqueductal grey matter and atrophy of mamillary bodies.*
➤ *Treatment: i.v. thiamine with a quick response, but 50% are left with a slow shuffling gait*
➤ *Always consider viral encephalitis (e.g. eastern equine, West Nile) with bilaterally symmetrical T2 hyperintense thalamic involvement with variable enhancement, or lymphoma with bilaterally symmetrical T2 hyperintensity with enhancement.*

REFERENCE
Ding J, *et al.* (2004). Alcohol intake and cerebral abnormalities on magnetic resonance imaging in a community-based population of middle-aged adults. *Stroke* 35:16–21.

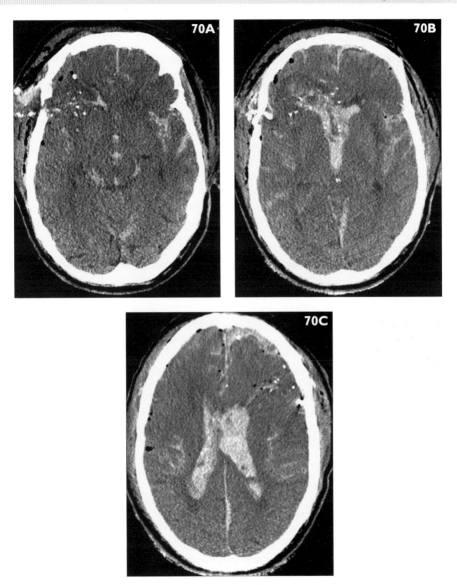

70 A patient presents after suffering an assault. Images **70A–C** are obtained.
i. What is the imaging modality of choice to evaluate gunshot injuries to the CNS?
ii. In single projectile gunshots, what is the most important bullet characteristic in terms of the amount of kinetic energy imparted to the target tissue?
iii. What is meant by calibre?

70: Answer

70 **DIAGNOSIS** Gunshot injury (pistol).

IMAGING FINDINGS Three axial noncontrast CT images (**70A–C**) demonstrate diffuse subarachnoid and intraventricular haemorrhage. A projectile track extends transversely from right to left across the frontal lobes. Multiple hyperdense bullet fragments are seen along the bullet course. Extensive hypoattenuating cerebral oedema is present throughout the frontal lobes bilaterally, both within and beyond the confines of the bullet track. A comminuted and mildly depressed skull fracture is present at the missile entry site on the right.

DIFFERENTIAL DIAGNOSIS This is a pattern of penetrating brain injury. It is important to note the extensive degree of haemorrhage and cerebral oedema. Haemorrhage may be due simply to parenchymal injury but a direct vascular injury should also be considered as the course of the bullet would have taken it in close proximity to the anterior cerebral arteries.

PATHOLOGY AND CLINICAL CORRELATION Gunshot injuries are an all-too-common finding in both urban and rural settings. When they are related to the brain, the results can be devastating. CT is the imaging modality of choice to evaluate such injuries (i). It is important to note that MRI is usually contraindicated in injuries in which metallic fragments remain within the central nervous system, even when the fragments are not ferromagnetic. Specific evaluation of entry and exit sites, intracranial fragments (bullet or bone), missile track (relation to vessels and ventricles), mass effect, and associated haemorrhage should be undertaken in all cases.

Primary injury to the brain is related to the ballistic properties of the bullet. The bullet itself crushes tissue in its path, creating a permanent track of tissue injury. More extensive damage is caused by cavitation and retraction due to energy transfer into the adjacent tissue. A bullet's kinetic energy is related to both mass and velocity ($KE = \frac{1}{2} mv^2$). However, since the available energy is related to the square of the velocity and only linearly related to the mass, velocity is usually the most important determinant of tissue injury with a single projectile bullet (ii). Other factors such as fragmentation and/or rotation of the bullet after impact also increase tissue injury and partially explain why exit wounds are most commonly larger than entry wounds.

A rudimentary understanding of guns/bullets is often helpful in discussions with emergency or trauma physicians. Rifle and handgun projectiles are described by their calibre which is a measure of the diameter of the bullet (iii). Calibre measurements can be expressed in either millimetres (e.g. 9 mm handgun) or inches (e.g. 0.44 magnum). Magnum refers to a load of extra power thus increasing bullet velocity. Handguns and rifles differ from shotguns in that shotguns simultaneously deliver multiple pellets with each shot. Shotgun loads are described by gauge, a measure inversely correlated with barrel diameter. Shotgun shells are varied and can contain anywhere from less than 10 to greater than 2,000 pellets. Close-range shotgun injuries are often devastating, as energy is transferred as in a single large fragmenting round.

TEACHING PEARLS

TEACHING PEARLS
➤ CT *is the modality of choice in evaluating gunshot injuries.*
➤ *Kinetic energy transfer causes extensive tissue damage beyond the track of the projectile.*

REFERENCES
Bartlett CS (2003). Clinical update: gunshot wound ballistics. *Clin Orthop* 408:28–57.
Marik PE, Varon J, Trask T (2002). Management of head trauma. *Chest* 122(2):699–711.

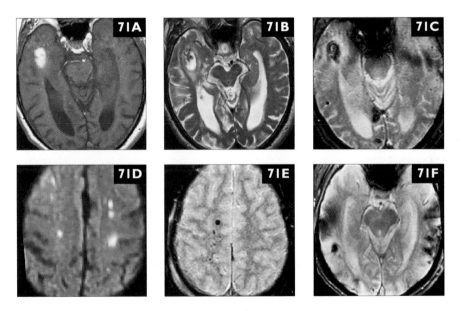

71 A 78-year-old male presents with memory loss occurring gradually over many years. The following images are obtained (**71A–C**).
i. Which sequences are shown?
ii. Where are the lesions located?
iii. What does the signal characteristics on images **71A, C** tell you about the lesions?
iv. What is the differential diagnosis of these multifocal lesions?
v. What other abnormality is visible in these images?

DIFFERENTIAL DIAGNOSIS Images 71D–F.

71: Answer

71 DIAGNOSIS Cerebral amyloid angiopathy (CAA), complicated by haemorrhage.

IMAGING FINDINGS Images 71A–C (axial T1, axial T2, and axial gradient echo, respectively) (i) demonstrate a T1/T2 hyperintense lesion in the right temporal lobe. These signal characteristics are typical for lesions containing blood products in a subacute stage (iii). This lesion is low in signal on the gradient echo image, reflecting susceptibility artifact that can be seen with blood products, metal, mineralization, or gas. The lesion with its surrounding oedema causes mass effect with effacement of the right temporal horn of the lateral ventricle. There is moderate diffuse (most likely age-related) volume loss (v). Additional foci of low signal are noted on the gradient echo sequence, particularly posteriorly in the occipital lobes (ii).

DIFFERENTIAL DIAGNOSIS The differential diagnosis (iv) of multifocal hemispheric haemorrhagic lesions includes:
- CAA (71A–C).
- Metastasis (see Question 75).
- Hypertensive microhaemorrhages.
- Septic emboli (71D, DWI).
- Diffuse axonal injury (71E, axial gradient echo).
- Multiple cavernous malformations.
- Coagulopathy (71F, axial gradient echo).

Differential considerations in this case should be based on the patient's age and the appearance of the lesions. CAA is exclusively a disease of older patients, with many lesions that will be apparent only on susceptibility-sensitive imaging sequences like gradient echo; unlike in other entities on this list, one would not expect the lesions to enhance. Metastatic lesions may show a predilection for the grey/white junction, but the lesions would typically enhance. In younger patients with a history of immunosuppression, endocarditis, or intravenous drug abuse, multiple foci of restricted diffusion and haemorrhage may represent septic emboli (71D). Multiple foci of microhaemorrhage at the grey/white junction and in the corpus callosum could represent shear injury (diffuse axonal injury) in the setting of previous trauma (71E); diffusion-weighted images might reveal additional lesions. Underlying coagulopathy leading to parenchymal haemorrhage should also be considered (71F), although this would be unlikely to be multifocal or appear as multiple small lesions as would be expected with CAA.

PATHOLOGY AND CLINICAL CORRELATION CAA results from deposition of the eosinophilic, extracellular protein amyloid in the media and adventitia of small and medium-sized vessels of the superficial layers of the cerebral cortex and leptomeninges, with sparing of the deep grey nuclei. This causes fibrinoid degeneration and microaneurysms of the affected vessels leading to lobar or multifocal haemorrhages, typically at the grey/white matter junction of the convexity.

CAA is not associated with systemic amyloidosis. Patients are usually more than 60 years old, normotensive, and present with stroke-like symptoms in case of lobar haemorrhage or progressive chronic dementia in the case of multifocal microbleeds.

CAA is found in 85% of patients with Alzheimer disease, causes 1% of all strokes, and is the most common cause of spontaneous intracranial haemorrhage in patients over 60.

TEACHING PEARLS
- ➤ *CAA is the most common cause of spontaneous intracranial haemorrhage in the elderly.*
- ➤ *Gradient echo images are exquisitely sensitive to the susceptibility artifact of microhaemorrhages associated with CAA and cavernous haemangiomas.*
- ➤ *Patients are typically demented and normotensive.*
- ➤ *CAA is the cause of lobar (rather than basal ganglia) haemorrhage.*
- ➤ *Patient age and medical history are important in finding the cause of intracranial haemorrhage.*

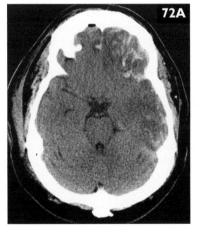 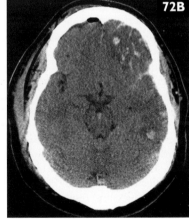

72 A patient presents after a fall from a horse, and the following images are obtained (72A, B).

i. Why are post-traumatic haemorrhages often seen involving the inferior aspect of the frontal and temporal lobes?

ii. Are findings always seen on initial scans?

iii. How do intracranial pressure and cerebral blood flow relate?

72 DIAGNOSIS Haemorrhagic contusion.

IMAGING FINDINGS Two axial images from a nonenhanced CT scan (**72A, B**) reveal parenchymal oedema and hyperdense haemorrhage, primarily involving the inferior left frontal and temporal lobes. Minimal haemorrhage is also seen within the parenchyma of the inferior medial right frontal lobe and the subarachnoid space of several frontal sulci and the interpeduncular fossa. A small amount of intracranial air is present anteriorly on the right and is related to a fracture through the frontal sinus (not included in these images).

DIFFERENTIAL DIAGNOSIS This diffuse pattern of haemorrhage, particularly with a history of trauma, suggests post-traumatic haemorrhagic contusion. If no history of trauma were present, haemorrhagic encephalitis could be considered.

PATHOLOGY AND CLINICAL CORRELATION Traumatic brain injury (TBI) is a major cause of disability and death in most Western nations and consumes an estimated $100 billion annually in the United States alone. Motor vehicle accidents are the most common cause of closed head injury, followed closely by falls. Haemorrhagic contusions are often seen along the inferior surfaces of the frontal and temporal lobes due to shearing motion of the brain and the relatively irregular osseous floor of the anterior and middle cranial fossa (**i**). Unfortunately, contusions are not always present on initial scan and can 'bloom' over the first 24–48 hr postinjury (**ii**). Therefore, patients with significant head trauma should be closely monitored and re-imaged if there is any decline in clinical status.

Patients should also be monitored for signs of increasing intracranial pressure and hydrocephalus. Secondary brain injury can occur due to neuronal damage caused by the physiologic response to the initial injury. Multiple substances have been implicated in initiating chemical cascades resulting in cell membrane breakdown and ionic shifts. However, one of the most important causes of secondary injury is hypoxia. In the post-traumatic state, global cerebral oedema or marked hydrocephalus can overwhelm the mechanisms of homeostasis and cause an increase in intracranial pressure, resulting in a decrease in cerebral blood flow and resultant hypoxia (**iii**).

TEACHING PEARLS
➤ *Haemorrhagic contusions are not always present on initial CT scans and can appear over the first 24–48 hr post-trauma.*
➤ *Trauma patients should be monitored for signs of increasing intracranial pressure.*

REFERENCES
Marik PE, Varon J, Trask T (2002). Management of head trauma. *Chest* **122**(2):699–711.
Marmarou A, *et al.* (2000). Contribution of oedema and cerebral blood volume to traumatic brain swelling in head-injured patients. *J Neurosurg* **93**(2):183–93.

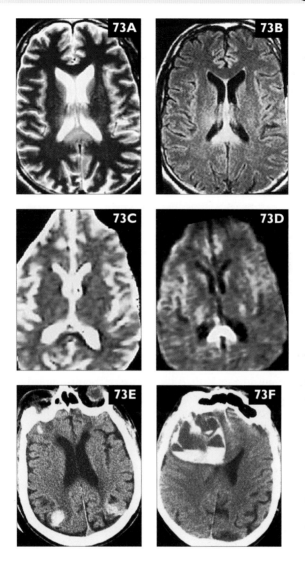

73 A 27-year-old female presents with loss of consciousness after a multiple vehicle accident, and the following images are obtained (73A–D).
i. Which sequences are shown?
ii. Where is the lesion located?
iii. What do 73C, D tell you about the morphology of the lesion?

DIFFERENTIAL DIAGNOSIS Images 73E, F.

73 **DIAGNOSIS** Diffuse axonal injury (DAI).

IMAGING FINDINGS Images **73A–D** (axial T2, axial FLAIR, axial gradient echo, and DWI, respectively) (**i**) demonstrate a T2 and FLAIR hyperintense lesion affecting the splenium of the corpus callosum (**ii**). The gradient echo image depicts susceptibility effect due to hemosiderin and DWI reveals restricted diffusion within the lesion (**iii**).

DIFFERENTIAL DIAGNOSIS The differential diagnosis of focal parenchymal lesions status post trauma includes:
- Coup/contrecoup (73E, axial unenhanced CT).
- Contusion (73F, axial unenhanced CT).
- DAI (73A–D).
- Internal carotid artery (ICA) dissection (see Question **46**).

Image **73E** shows a typical distribution of 'coup' lesion at the site of impact in the right frontal lobe (associated with calvarial fracture of the right orbital rim seen on bone windows, not shown) and two contrecoup lesions opposite the site of impact in the occipital lobes. Image **73F** demonstrates haemorrhagic contusion in the right frontal lobe with blood–fluid levels, right hemispheric oedema, and midline shift to the left. ICA dissection leads to parenchymal lesions only secondarily, due to infarcts; consider this lesion particularly when cortical infarcts are present in a typical vascular distribution in a younger patient.

PATHOLOGY AND CLINICAL CORRELATION DAI is caused by axonal stretching in the setting of trauma with high acceleration/deceleration and rotational forces. The overlying cortex moves at a different speed in relation to underlying white matter (WM), resulting in axonal shearing. Haemorrhage is the result of torn penetrating vessels. Because only 20% of lesions are haemorrhagic and visible, radiologists see only the 'tip of the iceberg': imaging findings are less severe than the clinical symptoms would suggest.

TEACHING PEARLS
- *Consider DAI in patient status post high-velocity trauma with clinical symptoms disproportionate to imaging findings.*
- *Despite a normal CT and MR, gradient echo susceptibility-weighted images should be ordered if DAI is suspected due to increased sensitivity for lesion detection.*
- *Multifocal small haemorrhagic foci occur at the grey/WM junction with prevalence of the frontotemporal lobes and lesions of the corpus callosum.*
- *DWI is also a useful imaging sequence for detecting lesions of DAI.*

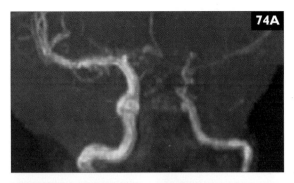

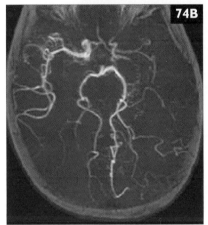

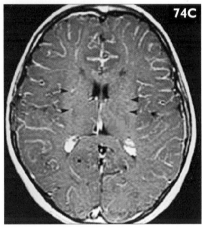

74 A 7-year-old female with a history of neurofibromatosis type 1 (NF1) presents with recurrent transient ischaemic attacks.

i. Which sequences are shown (74A–C)?

ii. What are the causes of this abnormality?

iii. What is the explanation of the sulcal enhancement seen in 74C?

74: Answer

74 DIAGNOSIS Moyamoya.

IMAGING FINDINGS 3D-TOF MRA (**74A, B**) (**i**) show severe narrowing of the left distal ICA, ACA, and MCA with compensatory enlargement of lenticulostriate and thalamostriate collaterals. Contrast-enhanced T1 image (**74C**) shows bright sulci due to leptomeningeal enhancement, the so called 'ivy sign', due to slow-flowing engorged pial vessels and thickened arachnoid membrane (**iii**).

DIFFERENTIAL DIAGNOSIS The MRA findings are compatible with Moyamoya ('puff of smoke' in Japanese), an idiopathic (Moyamoya disease) or acquired (Moyamoya syndrome) narrowing of the distal ICA and proximal circle of Willis vessels, with collateralization via lenticulostriate and thalamostriate perforators, as well as pial collaterals, first described on conventional angiography. Causes include idiopathic Moyamoya disease, which may have a genetic predisposition (about 10% familial), or any number of disorders associated with Moyamoya syndrome, including the phakomatoses (such as NF1), radiation therapy, sickle cell disease, certain drugs, prothrombotic states, vasculopathies, and basal meningitis (such as tuberculosis). There is also an association with other inherited disorders such as Down syndrome and tuberous sclerosis. See also Question **50** for the differential diagnosis of diffuse subarachnoid enhancement, which is observed here due to slow flow through the pial convexity vessels.

PATHOLOGY AND CLINICAL CORRELATION Moyamoya is a term that refers to the 'puff of smoke' angiographic pattern seen with progressive chronic occlusion of the distal ICA and proximal circle of Willis as in this case (**ii**). Children present with transient ischaemic attacks, whereas adults present with intracranial haemorrhage.

TEACHING PEARLS
> *Look for multiple punctate enhancing foci on contrast-enhanced CT (CECT), or flow voids on unenhanced MR in the basal ganglia, representing enlarged collateral vessels.*
> *Children present with transient ischaemic attacks, whereas adults present with subarachnoid and intraventricular haemorrhage.*

REFERENCES
Fujisawa I, *et al.* (1987). Moyamoya disease: MR imaging. *Radiology* **164**:103–5.
Osborn AG, *et al.* (2004). *Brain*. Amirsys, Salt Lake City, Chapter I-4, pp. 42–5.
Sucholeiki R, Chawla J (2006). Moyamoya disease. eMedicine, last updated November 2006.

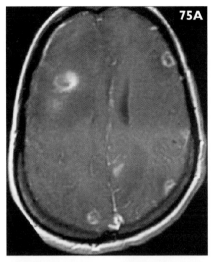

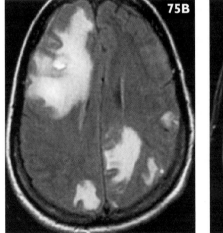
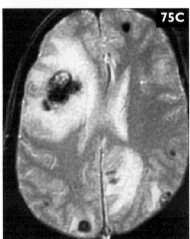

75 A 67-year-old male presents with known intracranial haemorrhage detected with CT.

i. What sequences are shown (75A–C)?

ii. What is the differential diagnosis?

75 **Diagnosis** Metastatic malignant melanoma.

Imaging findings Images 75A–C (axial contrast-enhanced T1, axial FLAIR, and axial gradient echo susceptibility sequence, respectively [i]) demonstrate multiple enhancing lesions associated with extensive parenchymal oedema. Gradient echo images show that each of these lesions is associated with susceptibility artifact ('black holes') due to underlying haemorrhage (acute phase due to deoxyhaemoglobin, chronic phase due to hemosiderin).

Differential diagnosis The differential diagnosis of multifocal hemispheric haemorrhagic lesions – which depends on patient age, anatomic distribution, and chronicity – includes cerebral amyloid angiopathy (elderly, peripheral cortical), metastasis (adult), hypertensive microhaemorrhages (deep cortical), septic emboli (heterogeneous), diffuse axonal injury (post traumatic, brainstem and grey/white regions), multiple cavernous malformations (wide range of ages and anatomic regions), and coagulopathy (varies). The differential also clearly depends on the patient's specific history (such as a history of previous malignancy, as in this case, or hypertension) (ii).

Pathology and clinical considerations Metastatic disease must always be a consideration when encountering enhancing adult intraparenchymal lesions. Lesions are classically located at the grey–white matter interface and can vary in size and number. Patients present with acute onset neurological symptoms related to the acute haemorrhagic event. Primary tumours that are particularly associated with haemorrhage are given by the 'MR/CT' mnemonic: melanoma, renal cell carcinoma, choriocarcinoma, and thyroid carcinoma. However, given its overall prevalence, lung cancer may be the most common cause of a haemorrhagic metastasis.

Teaching pearls
> *Parenchymal intracranial haemorrhage is seen in 3–14% of metastases; the cell types most likely to bleed are given by the 'MR/CT' mnemonic described above, although statistically lung cancer may be the most common cause.*
> *Multiple diffusely spread lesions occur at grey/white matter junctions with different size and marked oedema.*
> *In the setting of parenchymal haemorrhage, it can be difficult to determine if there is an underlying lesion (such as metastasis or a vascular malformation). Look for irregular patterns of enhancement or haemorrhage. Follow-up imaging that allows resolution of the acute changes of haemorrhage can be a useful adjunct to exclude an underlying lesion.*

References
Fazekas F, *et al.* (1999). Histopathologic analysis of foci of signal loss on gradient-echo T2* -weighted MR images in patients with spontaneous intracranial hemorrhage. *AJNR* 20:637–42.
Osborn AG, *et al.* (2004). *Brain*. Amirsys, Salt Lake City, Chapter I-6, pp. 140–3.

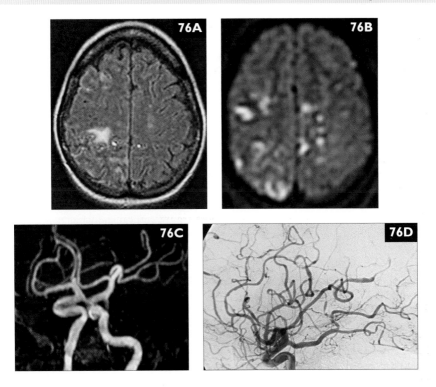

76 A 63-year-old patient presents with hemiparesis. The following images are obtained (76A–D).

i. Does this process affect cortical grey matter, subcortical white matter, or both?

ii. Are infarcts limited to a single vessel distribution?

iii. What is the angiographic pattern demonstrated in image 76D?

76: Answer

76 DIAGNOSIS CNS vasculitis.

IMAGING FINDINGS FLAIR image (76A) demonstrates multifocal regions of increased T2 signal within the cortical grey and subcortical white matter bilaterally (i). Trace diffusion-weighted image (76B) shows increased signal representing restricted diffusion within a similar distribution (though not shown, ADC map confirmed true diffusion-restriction). Note that cortical infarcts are seen in both the anterior and posterior circulation bilaterally, encompassing several vascular distributions (ii). Three-dimensional noncontrast time-of-flight MRA focused on the anterior circulation (76C) demonstrates diffuse irregularity of vessel lumen contour with multifocal regions of vascular stenosis. This vascular 'beading' is confirmed by conventional angiography (76D) (iii).

DIFFERENTIAL DIAGNOSIS Multifocal patchy regions of cortical and white matter signal abnormality without mass effect is a nonspecific finding raising many differential considerations. Chronic microvascular disease secondary to atherosclerosis (with or without associated cortical infarcts) is the most common cause, but vasculitis should be always be considered when the distribution is more peripheral, especially in younger patients. Angiography demonstrates a typical beaded pattern of alternating stenoses and regions of vascular dilatation when vasculitis affects the large or medium sized vessels of the cerebral circulation, but can be normal when only the small vessels are involved. Therefore, a negative angiogram does not exclude the diagnosis. When angiographic findings are present, narrowing tends to be circumpherential, differentiating this process from the primarily eccentric narrowing seen with atherosclerosis.

PATHOLOGY AND CLINICAL CORRELATION Vasculitis refers to a heterogeneous group of clinicopathological disorders that cause inflammation of blood vessels. Many causes are immune-modulated. Untreated, CNS vasculitis leads to a variety of clinical neurological manifestations related to ischaemia and, ultimately, to infarction. Multiple systems have been devised in order to group the many causes of vasculitis. One of the most basic systems divides vasculitides into infectious and noninfectious causes. Infectious causes can be due to a variety of pathogens including many viral, bacterial, and fungal infections. Noninfectious aetiologies are even more varied and can be subdivided into systemic disorders (polyarteritis nodosa, Wegeners, giant cell arteritis, systemic lupus erythematosus), paraneoplastic origin (often preceding detection of the primary neoplasm), drug-related (prescription and 'street' drugs), and granulomatous angiitis (primary angiitis of the CNS).

Though the diagnosis can be suggested by radiographic and laboratory findings, definitive diagnosis is often made only after brain biopsy. Treatment involves addressing the specific cause, though steroids and immunosuppressive agents are often administered.

TEACHING PEARLS
➤ *Vasculitis is inflammation of vessel walls due to any of a large number of causes.*
➤ *Definitive diagnosis often requires biopsy.*
➤ *Treatment is often by steroids and immunosuppressive agents.*

REFERENCES
Kadkhodayan Y, *et al.* (2004). Primary angiitis of the central nervous system at conventional angiography. *Radiology* **233**(3):878–82.
Younger DS (2004). Vasculitis of the nervous system. *Curr Opin Neurol* **17**:317–336.

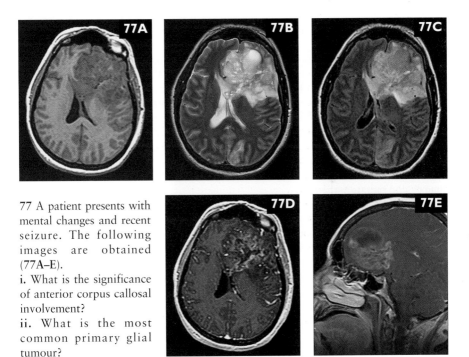

77 A patient presents with mental changes and recent seizure. The following images are obtained (77A–E).

i. What is the significance of anterior corpus callosal involvement?

ii. What is the most common primary glial tumour?

iii. Can the margin of neoplastic cells be clearly defined in primary CNS neoplasms?

77 DIAGNOSIS Glioblastoma multiforme (GBM).

IMAGING FINDINGS T1- and T2-weighted images (**77A, B**) reveal a large heterogeneous mass centred within the left frontal lobe containing both solid and cystic components. FLAIR sequence (**77C**) better demonstrates abnormal signal associated with the mass crossing the midline within the anterior corpus callosum. Postcontrast axial and sagittal T1 images (**77D, E**) show diffuse heterogeneous enhancement within the solid portions of the mass.

Subtle cortical T2 hyperintensity is also present within the medial left occipital pole due to a subacute infarction.

DIFFERENTIAL DIAGNOSIS In isolation, an intracranial mass raises a large number of differential considerations. The fact that this lesion shows signal crossing the midline is of considerable significance and severely narrows the differential diagnosis (**i**). In general, GBM, lymphoma, and occasionally demyelination or infection cross the corpus callosum. History can occasionally aid in limiting this differential further.

PATHOLOGY AND CLINICAL CORRELATION GBM is an aggressive WHO grade 4 glial tumour with extremely poor prognosis. Unfortunately, these are the most common primary brain tumour and affect all age groups (**ii**). GBMs can form de novo or can progress from malignant degeneration of lower grade tumours. Central necrosis and cystic change are common findings but need not be present. Tumours progress rapidly with a mean survival time measured in months. It is important to realize that neoplastic cells extend far beyond enhancing margins and even the area of T2 abnormality (**iii**). No treatment is completely effective in arresting progression, but tumours are often surgically debulked and subsequently treated with combined chemo- and radiation therapy.

TEACHING PEARLS
➤ *GBMs are aggressive infiltrating masses often containing central necrosis.*
➤ *These tumours are essentially universally fatal and have mean survival times of only several months.*
➤ *GBM along with lymphoma and occasionally infection or demyelination can infiltrate the fibres of the corpus callosum.*

REFERENCES
Atlas SW (1990). Adult supratentorial tumours. *Semin Roentgenol* **25**:130–54.
Earnest F IV, *et al* (1988). Cerebral astrocytomas: histopathologic correlation on MR and CT contrast enhancement with stereotactic biopsy. *Radiology* **166**:823–7.
Lacroix M, *et al.* (2001). A multivariate analysis of 416 patients with GBM: prognosis, extent of resection, and survival. *J Neurosurg* **95**:190–8.

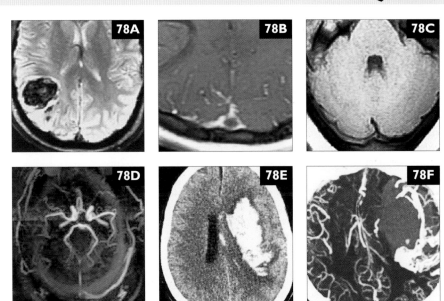

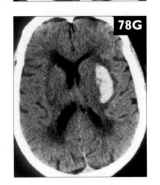

78 A 35-year-old female presents with seizures and vomiting, and the following images are obtained (78A–D).

i. Which sequences are shown?

ii. What is the name of the sign demonstrated in 78B?

iii. What are the findings on images 78C, D?

iv. How are the findings in 78B–D associated with the mass in 78A?

DIFFERENTIAL DIAGNOSIS Images 78E–G.

78: Answer

78 DIAGNOSIS Dural sinus thrombosis and cortical venous thrombosis (DST/CVT), complicated by parenchymal haemorrhage.

IMAGING FINDINGS Images **78A–D** (axial gradient echo, axial contrast enhanced T1, axial T1, and MR venography [MRV], respectively) **(i)** demonstrate parenchymal haemorrhage in the right parietal lobe, causing susceptibility effect on gradient echo images. This is a haemorrhagic venous infarct. Image **78B** shows the 'empty delta' sign **(ii)** with a hypointense clot in the superior sagittal sinus surrounded by enhancing dura. In addition, acute T1 isointense thrombus in the right transverse sinus is seen, resulting in absence of flow in the MRV (**78C, D**) **(iii)**.

DIFFERENTIAL DIAGNOSIS The differential diagnosis of focal intraparenchymal nontraumatic haemorrhage includes:
- Hypertension (**78G**, axial unenhanced CT).
- Cerebral amyloid angiopathy.
- Haemorrhagic infarction.
- Neoplasm.
- Ruptured aneurysm (see Question **81**).
- Arteriovenous malformation (AVM) (**78E, F**, axial unenhanced CT and coronal CT angiography [CTA] reformat).
- Cavernous malformation.
- Coagulopathy.

Determining the cause of parenchymal haemorrhage can present a clinical dilemma: it is important to consider the possibility of venous haemorrhagic infarct especially when the haemorrhage is in an unusual location or an infarct does not correspond to usual vascular territories. In some cases, it can be difficult to exclude an underlying neoplasm or vascular abnormality. Images **78E, F** depict a large haemorrhagic lesion in the right hemisphere representing an AVM, with enlarged feeding and draining vessels revealed by CTA. The basal ganglia haemorrhage in **78G** is typical of hypertension.

PATHOLOGY AND CLINICAL CORRELATION The most common cause for DST and CVT is factor V Leiden mutation, with a resistance to activated protein C. The association between DST, CVT, and venous infarction is the following: the thrombus initially forms in the dural sinus, propagates into cortical veins, and causes venous obstruction with infarction and, occasionally, haemorrhage **(iv)**.

TEACHING PEARLS
➤ *Haemorrhagic venous infarct is the most common cause for intracranial haemorrhage in infants.*
➤ *Empty delta sign can suggest thrombus in the superior sagittal sinus.*
➤ *Acute clot is hyperdense on unenhanced CT.*
➤ *Predisposing causes: pregnancy, oral contraceptives, dehydration, cirrhosis.*
➤ *Symptoms: headache, vomiting, seizures.*

REFERENCES (CASE 78)

Gibbs GF, *et al.* (2004). Improved image quality intracranial aneurysm. *Stroke* 35:372–4.

Grossman RI, *et al.* (2003). *Neuroradiology.* Mosby, Philadelphia, pp. 217–31.

Provenzale JM, Joseph GJ, Barboriak DP (1998). Dural sinus thrombosis: findings on CT and MR imaging and diagnostic pitfalls. *AJR* 170:770–83.

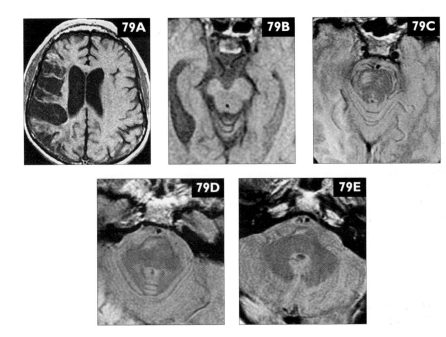

79 A patient presents with distant right hemispheric infarct. The following images are obtained (79A–E).

i. Which vessel was compromised resulting in the large right-sided infarction seen in image **79A**?

ii. What structure is severely atrophied in image **79B**?

iii. Describe the course of the corticospinal tracts.

79 DIAGNOSIS Wallerian degeneration.

IMAGING FINDINGS T1-weighted axial image (**79A**) reveals encephalomalacia and volume loss in the right middle cerebral artery (MCA) distribution, consistent with the patient's history of remote prior infarct (**i**). Proton density axial images show a small right cerebral peduncle (**79B**) and increased signal intensity coursing along the route of the corticospinal tracts into the ventral pons and medulla (**79C–E**) (**ii**).

DIFFERENTIAL DIAGNOSIS Abnormally increased T2 signal in the deep white matter tracts of the cerebral hemispheres and/or brainstem is a common finding that can be caused by a myriad of disease processes. However, if the signal is found to correspond to specific tracts (in this case the corticospinal), care should be taken to evaluate the cortex associated with that particular tract. If there is a cortical abnormality such as infarct or mass, the diagnosis of wallerian degeneration is readily made.

PATHOLOGY AND CLINICAL CORRELATION Wallerian degeneration is a well known process characterized by antegrade degeneration of axons due to death of neurons or proximal axons. It most commonly involves the corticospinal tract ipsilateral to an infarct in the MCA distribution. The corticospinal tract arises at the cortex and travels inferiorly via the centrum semiovale and corona radiata to converge primarily in the posterior limb of the internal capsule. It then travels in the anterior aspect of the cerebral peduncles before descending in the ventromedial pons to the medullary pyramids where 90% of the fibres cross midline (**iii**). This process can also occur in association with tumours, haemorrhage, vascular malformations, idiopathic movement disorders, and primary white matter disorders such as adrenoleukodystrophy and multiple sclerosis. The process induces essentially no inflammatory response.

MRI demonstrates increased T2 signal as early as 4–6 weeks following the initiating event. Abnormal MR signal is initially due to increased intracellular water content but permanent changes are secondary to gliosis. Conversely, CT shows only endstage changes such as atrophy of the midbrain and brainstem ipsilateral to the insult. There is no treatment.

TEACHING PEARLS
➤ *Wallerian degeneration is antegrade degeneration of axons due to death of associated neurons or proximal axons.*
➤ *Essentially any insult to the brain can result in wallerian degeneration.*

REFERENCES
Castillo M, Mukherji SK (1999). Early abnormalities related to postinfarction wallerian degeneration: evaluation with MR diffusion-weighted imaging. *J Comput Assist Tomog* 23(6):1004–7.
Liebeskind DS (2004). Wallerian degeneration of the corticospinal tracts. *Neurology* 62(5):828.

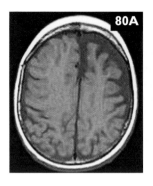 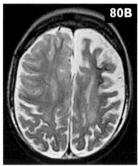 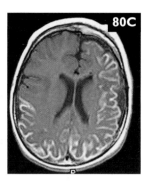

80 A 1-year-old child presents with infantile spasms, and the following images are obtained (80A–C).
i. Do the cerebral hemispheres appear of similar size?
ii. What white matter signal change do you see on the axial T2-weighted image (80B)?
iii. What does the postcontrast T1-weighted image (80C) show?
iv. What is the diagnosis?

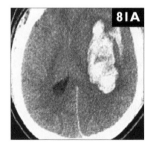 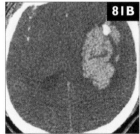 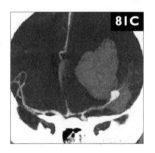

81 A 42-year-old female presents with acute onset hemiplegia.
i. Which sequences are shown (81A–C)?
ii. Could the location of the abnormality seen in 81C have been predicted by the location of haemorrhage?

80 **DIAGNOSIS** Sturge–Weber syndrome (bilateral) (**iv**).

IMAGING FINDINGS The extent of leptomeningeal angiomatosis is best demonstrated on T1-weighted postcontrast imaging, where it is seen as enhancement overlying gyri and filling sulci (**iii**). The underlying brain shows calcification of the cortex and subcortical white matter, best seen on CT, and T2 hypointensity (**ii**), likely effects of chronic venous ischaemia. The ipsilateral hemisphere eventually becomes atrophic (**i**: in this case left is smaller than right due to wider disease involvement). The choroid plexus may be enlarged due to hyperplasia, seen on the side ipsilateral to the side of the angioma. Choroidal angiomas may be seen as crescentic enhancement of the posterior globe.

PATHOLOGY AND CLINICAL CORRELATION Sturge–Weber syndrome causes angiomas of the face (port wine stain), choroid of eye, and leptomeninges. The intracranial angiomas predominately comprise a tangle of multiple capillaries and small veins on the brain surface. Patients commonly present with seizures and may have associated hemiparesis/anopsia or mental retardation.

TEACHING PEARL
➤ *Contrast MRI best depicts the extent of leptomeningeal angiomatosis.*

81 **DIAGNOSIS** Ruptured distal middle cerebral artery (MCA) aneurysm.

IMAGING FINDINGS Image **81A** (unenhanced CT) demonstrates large parenchymal haemorrhage in the left frontal lobe (basal ganglia, corona radiata) and subarachnoid haemorrhage in the left Sylvian fissure. Image **81B** is a contrast-enhanced source image from the CT angiography (CTA) dataset at the same level, and **81C** is the coronal reformatted CTA maximum intensity projection (MIP) image showing the left MCA aneurysm at an M2 branch beyond the MCA bifurcation (**i**).

DIFFERENTIAL DIAGNOSIS The differential diagnosis of focal intraparenchymal nontraumatic haemorrhage in this location depends on the patient's age and the clinical history, and includes hypertension, cerebral amyloid angiopathy, haemorrhagic infarction, underlying neoplasm, ruptured aneurysm, arteriovenous malformation (AVM), cavernous malformation, and parenchymal haemorrhage due to coagulopathy.

PATHOLOGY AND CLINICAL CORRELATION Intracranial aneurysms are round or lobulated arterial outpouchings of the intracranial arteries. Subarachnoid haemorrhage is the most common presenting event, often presenting as an acute onset, extremely severe headache (classically the 'worst headache of my life'). The majority are located in the anterior circulation and most arise from the circle of Willis. Risk of rupture depends on size (especially if greater than 10 mm) and morphology. Treatment can be either surgical or endovascular, depending on morphology, location, size, size of neck, multiplicity, and patient preference.

TEACHING PEARLS
➤ *Location of haemorrhage can localize the aneurysm: interhemispheric subarachnoid haemorrhage is associated with anterior communicating artery aneurysm and haemorrhage in the Sylvian fissure is associated with rupture of MCA bifurcation aneurysm (ii).*
➤ *CTA should be considered in the workup of any subarachnoid haemorrhage, despite atypical location or traumatic history.*
➤ *Although ruptured aneurysms more often result in subarachnoid haemorrhage, they can also present as intraparenchymal haemorrhage.*
➤ *Rupture risk is increased if:*
  ➤ *Multilobulated, rather than a round shape.*
  ➤ *Apical bleb is present.*
  ➤ *Aspect ratio (length/neck) is >1.6.*

REFERENCES
Grossman RI, *et al.* (2003). *Neuroradiology.* Mosby, Philadelphia, USA, pp. 217–31.
Osborn AG, *et al.* (2004). *Brain.* Amirsys, Salt Lake City, Chapter I-3, pp. 12–15.

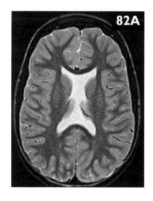 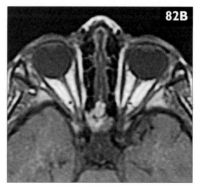

82 A patient presents with developmental delay and nystagmus. The following images are obtained (**82A, B**).
i. What normal structure is missing in the first image?
ii. What is the most common structural brain abnormality associated with this syndrome?

82 **DIAGNOSIS** Septo-optic dysplasia (SOD).

IMAGING FINDINGS The axial T2-weighted image (**82A**) demonstrates absence of the septum pellucidum (**i**). A high resolution axial T1-weighted image through the orbits (**82B**) reveals diminutive optic nerves bilaterally.

DIFFERENTIAL DIAGNOSIS The combination of absent septum pellucidum and small optic nerves is indicative of septo-optic dysplasia. Often in this disorder, the optic nerve hypoplasia is very subtle (or not present at all). Therefore, the diagnosis should be considered any time there is absence of the septum.

PATHOLOGY AND CLINICAL CORRELATION Most patients with SOD present in infancy. The syndrome is actually a disorder of midline prosencephalic development. While most cases are sporadic, there is a familial form. The forebrain, eyes, olfactory bulbs, and pituitary gland can all be affected. Pituitary dysfunction is seen in approximately 50% of cases and can be severe. Visual deficiency is variable. Additional abnormalities are often present, with schizencephaly being most common (**ii**). Prognosis depends upon the number and type of associated abnormalities.

TEACHING PEARLS
➤ *SOD should be considered any time there is absence of the septum pellucidum.*
➤ *SOD is associated with many other structural anomalies, most commonly schizencephaly.*

REFERENCES
Campbell CL (2003). Septo-optic dysplasia: a literature review. *Optometry* **74**(7):417–26.
Miller SP, *et al.* (2000). Septo-optic dysplasia plus: a spectrum of malformations of cortical development. *Neurology* **54**:1701–3.

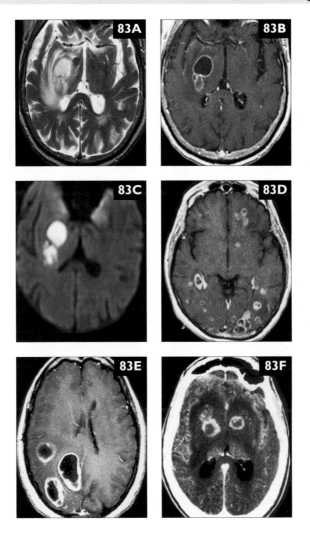

83 A 36-year-old male presents with headache, fever, increased erythrocyte sedimentation rate (ESR), and elevated white blood cell (WBC) count. The following images are obtained (83A–C).

i. Where are the lesions located?

ii. Describe the sequences and signal characteristics in 83A–C and the enhancement pattern in 83B.

iii. Which of these three sequences might be the most important in the differentiation from other entities with similar enhancement pattern?

DIFFERENTIAL DIAGNOSIS Images 83D–F.

83 DIAGNOSIS Pyogenic abscess.

IMAGING FINDINGS Images **83A–C** (axial T2, axial contrast-enhanced T1, and DWI, respectively) demonstrate a T2 hyperintense round lesion centred in the right thalamus and globus pallidus, surrounded by a hypointense rim and hyperintense oedema. The oedema extends laterally to the cortex of the insula and follows the optic radiation posteriorly. The oedema results in mass effect with effacement of the right Sylvian fissure (**i**). T1-weighted image after contrast administration (**83B**) depicts a well-defined enhancing rim, and DWI reveals restricted diffusion within the lesion (**ii**).

DIFFERENTIAL DIAGNOSIS The differential diagnosis of a ring-enhancing lesion includes:
- Glioblastoma multiforme.
- Multicentric glioma (**83E**, axial contrast-enhanced T1).
- Metastasis (**83D**, axial contrast-enhanced T1).
- Pyogenic abscess (**83A–C**).
- Neurocysticercosis (See Question **85**).
- Toxoplasmosis (**83F**, axial contrast-enhanced CT).
- Resolving haematoma.
- Contusion.
- Demyelination.
- Subacute infarct.

This is the classic differential of rim enhancement, known as MAGICDR (metastasis, abscess, glioma, infarct, contusion, demyelination, resolving haematoma). Other entities to consider when encountering a rim-enhancing lesion include neurocysticercosis, metastasis (**83D**) and mulicentric glioma (**83E**). The restricted diffusion of the lesion is the imaging feature that most favours abscess (**iii**). Another feature to evaluate is the appearance of the enhancing rim itself: neoplastic lesions (**83D, E**) usually have a thick, nodular, and irregular rim, while the inner rim is smooth. The opposite is seen in pyogenic abscesses. Toxoplasmosis (**83F**) should be considered in immunocompromised patients. The majority of toxoplasmosis lesions (75%) occur in the basal ganglia, while bacterial abscesses typically appear at the grey–white matter junction of the frontal and parietal lobes.

PATHOLOGY AND CLINICAL CORRELATION An abscess is defined as a focal pyogenic infection of the brain parenchyma due to bacterial, fungal, or parasitic infection. Typically an abscess is caused by:
- Haematogenous spread from an extracranial location, such as pulmonary, genitourinary, or cardiac (endocarditis).
- Direct extension from paranasal sinus, middle ear, or tooth infection.
- Penetrating trauma or surgery.
- In 25%, no identifiable source can be found.

An abscess may occur at any age and presents with headache, seizures, altered mental status change and/or focal neurological deficits. An increased ESR and WBC count complete the typical clinical setting. Primary treatment is drainage or excision of the abscess and steroids for limiting oedema. Antibiotics are used for primary therapy only, if the lesion is small (<2.5 cm) or in an early stage.

TEACHING PEARLS

➤ *Enhancing, T2 hypointense rim is suggestive of abscess. Classically, the rim is thinnest along the edge closest to the ventricle.*
➤ *Restricted diffusion within the abscess (DWI bright) is highly suggestive of abscess.*
➤ *Search for a local cause such as sinusitis, otitis media, or mastoiditis.*
➤ *Think of tuberculosis and toxoplasmosis in AIDS patients.*
➤ *Remember, a single rim enhancing mass in an adult most likely represents either metastasis or glioma, rather than infection.*

REFERENCES

Collazos J (2003). Opportunistic infections of the CNS in patients with AIDS: diagnosis and management. *CNS Drugs* **17**:869–87.
Guzman R, *et al.* (2002). Use of diffusion-weighted magnetic resonance imaging in differentiation purulent brain processes from cystic brain tumours. *J Neurosurg* **97**(5): 1101–7.
Zee CS, *et al.* (2000). Imaging of neurocysticercosis. *Neuroimaging Clin N Am* **10**(2):391–407.

---

84 A 2-year-old infant presents with diabetes insipidus, and the following image is obtained (**84**).
i. Where is the abnormality on this coronal enhanced T1 weighted image of the pituitary gland?
ii. What is your differential diagnosis? How does knowledge of the patient's age aid in ordering the differential?

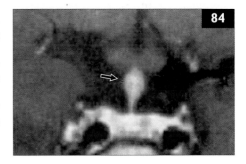

84 Diagnosis Langerhans cell histiocytosis.

Imaging findings Image 84 shows a vividly enhancing and thickened pituitary stalk (arrow) (i).

Differential diagnosis The differential diagnosis of pituitary stalk thickening or mass includes (ii):
- Langerhans cell histiocytosis (paediatric).
- Lymphoma (adult)/sarcoidosis (adult).
- Lymphocytic hypophysitis (pregnant female).
- Infection/abscess.
- Other neoplasm: metastases, germinoma (infants), glioma, PNET.
- Posterior pituitary ectopia.

Pathology and clinical correlation Langerhans cell histiocytosis (formerly called histiocytosis X) is a proliferative disorder of histiocytes that results in granuloma formation within multiple organ systems. The abnormality can either be isolated or diffuse. Typical abnormalities include osseous lesions (sharply marginated lytic skull lesions or involvement of the mastoid) and a thickened, enhancing pituitary infundibulum (as in this case). A rare manifestation is demyelination of the cerebellum. The infundibular lesion is most commonly associated with diabetes insipidus, although hypothalamic dysfunction or visual disturbance is also possible. Patients typically present before 2 years of age (ii).

Teaching pearls
➤ *Characterized by granulomas in any organ due to proliferation of Langerhans cell histiocytes.*
➤ *Lytic skull lesions and/or thick pituitary stalk in an infant/child are typical for histiocytosis; eosinophilic granuloma (EG) should be considered high in the differential diagnosis of any skull/facial bone lytic lesion in the paediatric age group.*
➤ *EG should be considered high in the differential diagnosis of any paediatric age patient presenting with diabetes insipidus.*

References
Kilborn TN, *et al.* (2003). Pediatric manifestations of Langerhans cell histiocytosis: a review of the clinical and radiological findings. *Clin Radiol* 58(4):269–78.
Meyer JS, *et al.* (1995). Langerhans cell histiocytosis: presentation and evolution of radiologic findings with clinical correlation. *Radiographics* 15:1135–46.

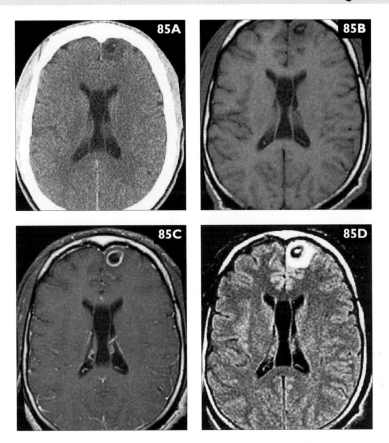

85 A 43-year-old female presents with altered mental status and the following images are obtained (85A–D).
i. Where is this lesion located?
ii. Describe the imaging findings.

85 **Diagnosis** Neurocysticercosis.

Imaging findings Images 85A–D (axial unenhanced CT, axial T1 MRI, axial post-contrast T1 MRI, and FLAIR MRI) demonstrate a CT hypodense, T1 MR hypointense, round cystic appearing lesion in the left superior frontal gyrus, surrounded by an enhancing well defined rim and moderate oedema, consistent with the colloidal vesicular stage of neurocysticercosis (**i, ii**). A hyperdense, hyperintense nodule within the lesion, best seen on the FLAIR sequence, represents the scolex of *Taenia solium* (pork tapeworm).

Differential diagnosis The broad differential diagnosis of a ring-enhancing lesion can be conveniently remembered using the 'MAGICDR' mnemonic (metastasis, abscess, glioma, infarct, contusion, demyelination, and resolving haematoma). Neurocysticercosis is an important additional consideration in this case, given the typical 'cyst with dot inside' appearance on FLAIR imaging. Prolonged resdience in an endemic region is an important historical clue to the diagnosis.

Pathology and clinical correlation Cysticercosis is an infection caused by the pork tapeworm, *Taenia solium*. The cysts associated with the infection are most commonly extra-axial, located in the subarachnoid space over the convexities, although lesion can also be seen in the basal cisterns and ventricles. Intraparenchymal lesions are usually located at the grey–white junction. There are four distinct stages of the infection each with a characteristic imaging appearance:
i.   Vesicular: thin walled cysts.
ii. Colloidal vesicular: hyperdense cysts on CT, with mild–severe surrounding oedema and enhancement on MR. The enhancing nodule is a scolex.
iii. Granular nodular: thickened cyst wall, decreased surrounding oedema.
iv. Nodular calcified: calcified lesions on CT, typically 'burned out' disease.

Teaching pearls
➤ *Cysticercosis is the most common parasitic infection in the world.*
➤ *Lesions can be located in the subarachnoid space over the convexities, the cerebral cisterns, the parenchyma, and the ventricles (in descending order of frequency).*
➤ *CNS infection is present in 60-90% of cysticercosis cases.*
➤ *Patients presents with seizures, headaches, and/or hydrocephalus.*

References
Collazos J (2003). Opportunistic infections of the CNS in patients with AIDS: diagnosis and management. *CNS Drugs* **17**:869–87.
Guzman R, *et al.* (2002). Use of diffusion-weighted magnetic resonance imaging in differentiation purulent brain processes from cystic brain tumours. *J Neurosurg* **97**(5): 1101–7.
Zee CS, *et al.* (2000). Imaging of neurocysticercosis. *Neuroimaging Clin N Am* **10**(2):391–407.

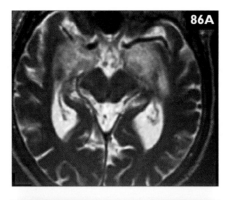

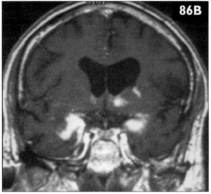

86 A 55-year-old male presents with mental status change and motor difficulties.
i. What is the abnormality (86A, B)?
ii. How does the bilaterally symmetrical appearance help to narrow the differential diagnosis?

86 **DIAGNOSIS** Lymphoma.

IMAGING FINDINGS Images 86A, B (axial T2 and coronal post contrast T1 MR image) demonstrate bilateral, multifocal, T2 hyperintense and homogenously enhancing lesions affecting the medial temporal lobes (symmetrical), thalami (slightly asymmetrical), and internal capsules bilaterally (i).

DIFFERENTIAL DIAGNOSIS The key factor in this case is the bilateral involvement of the temporal lobes. A limited differential diagnosis in this case is herpes simplex encephalitis, limbic encephalitis, and lymphoma. (See Question 54 for additional discussion.) More generally, a differential for primary CNS lymphoma includes toxoplasmosis, glioblastoma multiforme, abscess, and progressive multifocal leukoencephalopathy.

PATHOLOGY AND CLINICAL CORRELATION Lymphoma, along with the less common sarcoidosis, and unlike most other CNS pathologies, can present simultaneously in multiple different anatomical spaces (pachydural, leptomeningeal, intraparenchymal, skull) and, hence, has earned a reputation as the 'great mimic' in neuroradiology differential diagnosis. Deep grey nuclei, periventricular, and subependymal involvement is typical. Lymphoma should be strongly considered when there is multifocal or bilaterally symmetrical involvement (ii). The vast majority (98%) are B-cell non-Hodgkin lymphoma. Lesions are typically hyperdense on CT, relatively hyperintense on T1-weighted MRI, and hypointense on T2-weighted MRI, due to high nucleus-to-cytoplasm ratio. Lesions typically avidly enhance, although enhancement can be peripheral or heterogeneous in immunocompromised patients. Steroids can result in rapid resolution of the imaging abnormality, hence reducing the yield of biopsy.

TEACHING PEARLS
- *Lymphoma is hyperdense on CT, relatively hyperintense on T1-weighted MRI, and hypointense on T2-weighted MRI, due to high nucleus-to-cystoplasm ratio (a 'small round blue cell' tumour).*
- *Lesions typically enhance avidly, except in immunocompromised patients in whom the enhancement pattern can be peripheral or heterogeneous.*
- *Lymphoma, along with sarcoidosis, has become the 'great mimicker' in neuroradiology, as it can present simultaneously in any combination of multiple different CNS compartments (discussed above).*
- *Consider lymphoma when there are bilaterally symmetrical or multifocal enhancing masses.*

REFERENCE
Koeller KK, *et al.* (1997). Primary central nervous system lymphoma: radiologic-pathologic correlation. *Radiographics* **17**(6):1497–526.

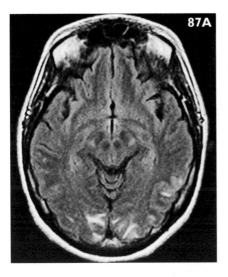

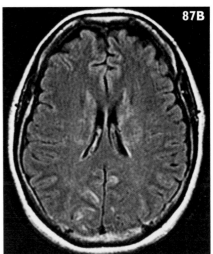

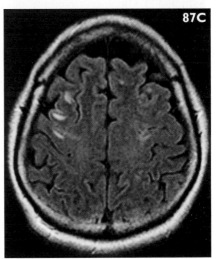

87 A 31-year-old pregnant female presents with eclampsia and seizure, and the following images are obtained (87A–C).

i. Are the areas of signal abnormality affecting cortical grey matter, subcortical white matter, or both?

ii. Are the findings primarily within an anterior or posterior distribution?

iii. What may happen if this entity is not recognized in a timely manner?

87 DIAGNOSIS Posterior reversible encephalopathy syndrome (PRES).

IMAGING FINDINGS Axial FLAIR images reveal generally symmetric hyperintense signal within the cortical grey and subcortical white matter of the occipital and posterior temporal lobes (**87A, B**) (**i**). Similar signal abnormality is present but is less pronounced within the posterior frontal lobes (**87C**). There was no associated enhancement or diffusion restriction (not shown).

DIFFERENTIAL DIAGNOSIS The differential diagnosis includes PRES, multifocal infarct, encephalitis, vasculitis, and low-grade tumour. The lack of diffusion restriction essentially rules out infarction. History can often aid in the diagnosis of PRES.

PATHOLOGY AND CLINICAL CORRELATION PRES classically consists of vasogenic oedema primarily within the posterior circulation (**ii**). Findings are generally symmetric and are typically within the cortex and subcortical white matter of the occipital and parietal lobes. These findings occur to a lesser degree in the posterior frontal and temporal lobes, the corona radiata, the pons, the cerebellum, and other locations. FLAIR images typically show the pathology best. PRES affects all age groups, with children showing greater vulnerability to the pathologic process.

The most common causes of PRES are hypertension, pre-eclampsia/eclampsia, ciclosporin A toxicity, and the uremic encephalopathies. There is resultant breakdown of the normal cerebral autoregulation either due to increased blood pressure or direct toxic effects upon the vascular endothelium. This process ultimately leads to leakage of fluids (and rarely red blood cells) into the interstitium, resulting in vasogenic oedema. There is no cytotoxic oedema in uncomplicated PRES and therefore no diffusion restriction.

Common presentations include headache, altered mental status, seizure, and visual loss. Though seizures are often associated with PRES, they are likely a result, rather than a cause, of the pathology. It is postulated that the findings are more commonly posterior due to the relatively sparse sympathetic innervation of the vertebrobasilar circulation (thus less ability to autoregulate). Findings were initially described in the subcortical white matter possibly because there is less cellular density in this region as compared to the adjacent cortex, thus allowing more space for the accumulation of oedema. It is now widely accepted that both regions are involved.

If the cause of PRES is addressed promptly, the symptoms and radiological abnormalities can be completely reversed. However, if unaddressed, the syndrome can progress to focal irreversible ischaemia and infarction (**iii**).

TEACHING PEARLS
➤ *PRES is most often caused by hypertension resulting in dysfunction of the normal cerebral vascular autoregulation.*
➤ *While findings are most common in the posterior distribution, they can be seen in almost all regions of the brain.*
➤ *If the cause of PRES is not addressed in a timely manner, PRES can progress to ischaemia and infarction.*

REFERENCES (CASE 87)

Casey SO, *et al.* (2000). Posterior reversible encephalopathy syndrome: Utility of fluid-attenuation inversion recovery MR imaging in the detection of cortical and subcortical lesions. *AJNR* **21**:1199–1206.

Covarrubias DJ, Luetmer PH, Campeau NG (2002) Posterior reversible encephalopathy syndrome: prognostic utility of quantitative diffusion-weighted MR images. *AJNR* **23**:1038–48.

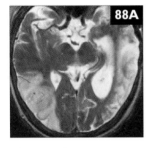
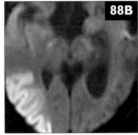
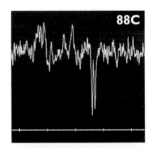

88 A 19-year-old male presents with sudden onset of headache, followed by hemianopsia and aphasia. The following images are obtained (**88A–C**).

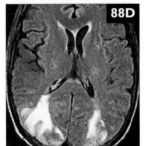
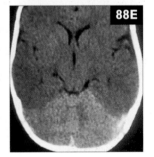

i. Which sequences are shown?
ii. What does signal and morphology of the lesion in image **88B** tell you?
iii. Is the lesion confined to a vascular territory?
iv. Which characteristic finding is shown in **88C**?

DIFFERENTIAL DIAGNOSIS Images 88D, E.

88 DIAGNOSIS Mitochondrial myopathy, encephalopathy, lactic acidosis, and stroke-like episodes (MELAS).

IMAGING FINDINGS Images 88A–C (axial T2, DWI, MR spectroscopy, respectively) (**i**) demonstrate an area of high signal in the right temporal and occipital lobe with gyral swelling and sparing of the medial occipital gyri. DWI reveals apparent restricted diffusion confined to the cortex (**ii**), in a distribution that does not match a typical vascular territory (**iii**). Spectroscopy shows a prominent inverted lactate peak at 1.3 ppm, typical for MELAS (**iv**).

DIFFERENTIAL DIAGNOSIS The differential diagnosis of a stroke-like posterior cerebral artery (PCA) territory lesion includes:
• Acute PCA infarct.
• Hypotensive stroke.
• Severe hypoglycaemia.
• Posterior reversible encephalopathy syndrome (PRES) (eclampsia) (see Question **99**).
• PRES (ciclosporin) (**88D**, axial FLAIR).
• Child abuse (**88E**, axial unenhanced CT).
• MELAS (**88A–C**).
• Acute cerebral hyperaemia (postictal, postcarotid endarterectomy).
• Acute demyelinating disease.
• Gliomatosis cerebri.
Image **88D** demonstrates bioccipital wedge-shaped hyperintense lesions affecting the cortex and white matter (WM) in a patient with PRES (see Question **99**) after ciclosporin therapy. Image **88E** shows hypodensity, oedema, sulcal effacement, and lack of grey–WM differentiation affecting the entire brain with sparing of the posterior circulation territory in a child following strangulation, which causes anoxic injury in the anterior circulation.

PATHOLOGY AND CLINICAL CORRELATION MELAS is an inherited disorder of mitochondrial energy production caused by point mutation in mitochondrial DNA. It is characterized by recurrent stroke-like episodes beginning in late childhood. The acute onset is often associated with headache, hemianopsia, and psychosis followed by stroke-like symptoms with hemiplegia and muscle weakness. Prognosis of MELAS is variable; however, patients in general tend to have poor outcome. The encephalomyopathy tends to progress to dementia. Currently, no therapies are effective.

TEACHING PEARLS
➤ *Think of MELAS in a teenager or young adult patient with recurrent stroke-like cortical lesions which cross vascular territories and appear, disappear, and reappear elsewhere.*
➤ *Acute imaging findings include: swollen gyri, compressed sulci, DWI-positive.*
➤ *Chronic imaging findings: progresive atrophy of basal ganglia and cerebral cortex, with multiple T2 hyperintense lesions of the basal ganglia and deep WM.*
➤ *MR spectroscopy shows a prominent lactate doublet.*
➤ *Mean age of onset is 15 years, with over 90% symptomatic by age 40.*

REFERENCES
Abe K, *et al.* (2004). Comparison of conventional and diffusion-weighted MRI and proton MR spectroscopy in patients with mitochondrial encephalomyopathy, lactic acidosis, and stroke-like events. *Neuroradiology* **46**(2):113–7.
Osborn AG, *et al.* (2004). *Brain.* Amirsys, Salt Lake City, Chapter I-10, pp. 28–31.

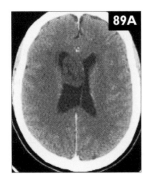 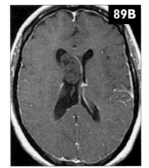 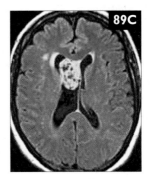

89 A 62-year-old male presents with a lesion noted incidentally on CT and MR (89A–C).
i. Where is the mass located?
ii. Describe the morphology and signal characteristics of the tumour.

89 **DIAGNOSIS** Subependymoma.

IMAGING FINDINGS Images 89A–C show a FLAIR hyperintense nonenhancing tumour with multiple intratumoural cysts in the frontal horn of the right lateral ventricle displacing the septum pellucidum to the left side (i).

DIFFERENTIAL DIAGNOSIS The differential diagnosis of masses located in the lateral ventricle or along the margin of the lateral ventricle is also presented in Question **98**. This differential includes central neurocytoma, subependymoma, and subependymal giant cell astrocytoma.

PATHOLOGY AND CLINICAL CORRELATION Subependymoma is a benign intraventricular tumour. The lesion is most commonly found in the 4th ventricle, with less common locations being the lateral and third ventricles. Lesions are T2 hyperintense and nonenhancing (ii). While most patients are asymptomatic, symptoms are possible if there is associated hydrocephalus or increased intracranial pressure. Surgery is curative.

TEACHING PEARLS
➤ *Subependymoma is a T2 hyperintense, lobular, nonenhancing, intraventricular mass.*
➤ *Most common location is the 4th ventricle (often expanding through the foramen of Magendie). Less common locations are the lateral and 3rd ventricles.*
➤ *Calcifications and cysts are common.*
➤ *Age peak: 5th to 6th decades, males more common than females.*

REFERENCES
Hoeffel C, *et al.* (1995) MR manifestations of subependymomas. *AJNR* **16**:2121–9.
Koeller KK, Sandberg GD (2002). From the Archives of the AFIP: cerebral intraventricular neoplasms: radiologic-pathologic correlation. *Radiographics* **22**:1473–505.

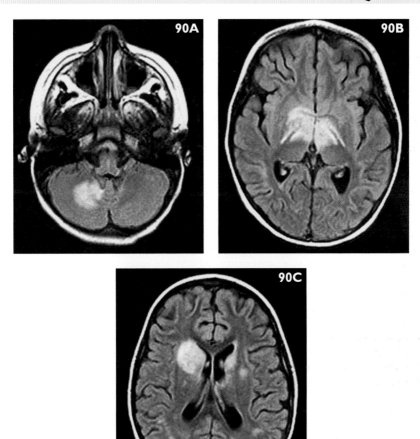

90 A young adult presents with seizure and decreased responsiveness 1 week after a viral upper respiratory infection. The following images are obtained (90A–C).

i. What is the most common postviral cerebral disorder?

ii. Is this process more common in a certain age group?

iii. Do clinical symptoms temporally correlate with imaging findings?

90 **DIAGNOSIS** Acute disseminated encephalomyelitis (ADEM).

IMAGING FINDINGS White matter disease.

DIFFERENTIAL DIAGNOSIS Differential diagnosis would primarily include vasculitis, multiple sclerosis (MS), viral encephalitis and, possibly, low-grade glial tumour. MRI findings suggesting ADEM rather than MS include involvement of the cortex, subcortical, and parieto-occipital periventricular white matter. MS lesions classically abut and extend transversely from the lateral ventricle ependymal lining (Dawson's fingers). ADEM lesions are commonly large with little mass effect, which can be confused with a low-grade glioma if there is a single lesion. Acute onset and history of preceding viral infection or immunization should suggest ADEM. Differentiation from vasculitis is often difficult when the lesions are peripheral and arteriograms are often performed for further evaluation. Contrast enhancement is variable and does not necessarily correlate with a worse clinical picture.

PATHOLOGY AND CLINICAL CORRELATION ADEM is a monophasic immune-mediated disorder affecting the myelin sheaths with relative sparing of the axons. Classical presentation is following viral infection or immunization but can be idiopathic. Though rare, ADEM is the most common postviral cerebral disorder (i). ADEM can affect any age group but is most commonly seen in children (ii). Onset is usually rapid, with the most common symptoms including lethargy, coma, seizure, hemiparesis, cranial nerve disorders, long tract signs, movement disorders, and/or behavioural changes. Cerebrospinal fluid (CSF) shows mildly elevated leukocytes and protein, which can make clinical differentiation from viral encephalitis difficult.

Prognosis is variable with 10–30% reported mortality and approximately 25% of patients left with residual neurologic sequelae. Imaging findings have been reported to lag behind clinical symptoms and improvement (iii). Most imaging findings completely resolve within months. Treatment is with IV or oral steroids.

Two rare subgroups of ADEM exist. Acute haemorrhagic encephalomyelitis (AHEM) is classically seen in young patients and shows a fulminant course often ending in death. As the name implies, there is haemorrhage from the cortical lesions and CSF erythrocytes are noted. The second variant is a biphasic form of the disorder occurring in up to 10% of patients, refereed to as biphasic disseminated encephalomyelitis (BDEM). Differentiation of this subset of disease from MS is controversial.

TEACHING PEARLS
➤ ADEM *is the most common postviral cerebral abnormality.*
➤ *Focal demyelinating lesions are seen on MRI and are classically bilateral and symmetric. Imaging findings resolve after resolution of symptoms.*
➤ *All age groups are affected.*

REFERENCES (CASE 90)

Honkaniemi J, *et al.* (2001). Delayed MR imaging changes in acute disseminated encephalomyelitis. *AJNR* **22**:1117–24.

Singh S, Alexander M, Korah, I (1999). Acute dissiminated encephalomyelitis: MR imaging features. *AJR* **173**:1101–7.

Tenenbaum S, Chamoles N, Fejerman N (2002). Acute disseminated encephalomyelitis: a long-term flow-up study of 84 pediatric patients. *Neurology* **59**(8):1224–31.

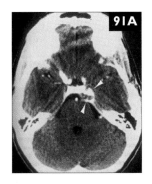
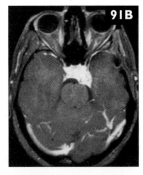
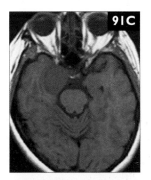

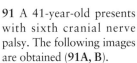
91 A 41-year-old presents with sixth cranial nerve palsy. The following images are obtained (**91A, B**).

i. Where is the lesion located?

ii. What is the most important differential diagnosis and how can the location help to distinguish the diagnosis?

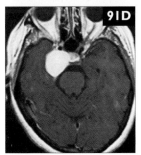
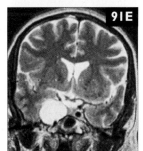

DIFFERENTIAL DIAGNOSIS Images 91C–E.

91 DIAGNOSIS Chondrosarcoma.

IMAGING FINDINGS Images **91A, B** (axial unenhanced CT and axial contrast-enhanced T1, respectively) demonstrate a densely calcified enhancing parasellar mass (arrowheads) arising from the left petroclival synchondrosis (i) and effacing the suprasellar and ambient cisterns.

DIFFERENTIAL DIAGNOSIS The differential diagnosis (ii) of a cavernous sinus region mass includes:
Dural:
• Meningioma (see Question 95).
• Sarcoidosis.
• Metastasis.
• Lymphoma.
• Perineural spread of tumour.
• Schwannoma.
• Aneurysm.
• Cavernous sinus cavernous haemangioma (**91C–E**, axial T1, axial T1 postcontrast, and coronal T2).
Osseus:
• Chordoma.
• Chondrosarcoma (**91A, B**).
• Plasmacytoma.
• Chondromyxoid fibroma.
• Osteogenic sarcoma.
• Jugular foramen lesions.
• Petrous apex lesions.
The differential diagnosis of parasellar masses includes lesions of bone, including the clivus and the petroclival synchondrosis. The classic differential diagnosis in this location for a bony lesion is chordoma (usually midline) versus chondrosarcoma (off-midline at the petroclival synchondrosis, as in this case). The other major differential consideration is lesion of the cavernous sinus, including lymphoma, meningioma, schwannoma, or aneurysm. Images **91C–E** show a T1 hypointense and T2 hyperintense homogenously enhancing right cavernous sinus mass with narrowing and inferior displacement of the cavernous segment of the ICA, representing a haemangioma. Cavernous haemangiomas are rarely found in an extracerebral location (ii); these uncommon lesions are seen in the cavernous sinus or cerebellopontine angles. They compromise about 1% of all parasellar masses.

PATHOLOGY AND CLINICAL CORRELATION The petroclival and spheno-occipital synchondrosis are sites in the mature skull that undergo endochondral ossification. It is hypothesized that islands of residual endochondral cartilage may be present in these areas and that chondrosarcomas develop from these chondrocytes. Most of these chondrosarcomas are well or moderately differentiated, local invasive, and rarely metastatic. Treatment is combined radical resection and radiation.

TEACHING PEARLS (CASE 91)

➤ *Chondrosarcoma is an off-midline mass arising from the petro-occipital (2/3) or spheno-occipital synchondrosis (1/3).*
➤ *It is a heterogenously enhancing tumour with arc or ring-like chondroid calcification (in 50%) and bone destruction (in 50%).*
➤ *The most important differential diagnosis is chordoma, which arise along the midline and are rarely if ever mineralized.*
➤ *Median patient age is 40 years.*

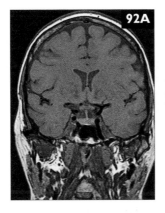

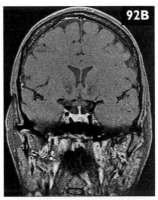

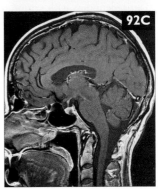

92 A patient presents with amenorrhea, and the following images are obtained (**92A–C**).

i. Describe the enhancement pattern of the normal pituitary gland.

ii. What size differentiates the two basic forms of primary pituitary tumours?

iii. Describe two ways in which sellar lesions can cause symptoms.

92 DIAGNOSIS Pituitary microadenoma.

IMAGING FINDINGS Thin section high resolution images are presented. Coronal nonenhanced T1 image shows no abnormality (**92A**). There is no superior contour abnormality of the pituitary gland. After contrast administration, there is a 7 mm focus of decreased enhancement seen within the posterior left aspect of the pituitary gland (**92A, B**). The pituitary stalk remains midline. There is no mass effect upon the optic chiasm.

DIFFERENTIAL DIAGNOSIS Nonenhancing solid pituitary lesions usually represent adenomas. On immediate postcontrast imaging, these tumours show relatively little enhancement compared to the normal homogenously enhancing gland (**i**). A tumour is termed a microadenoma if it is less than 1 cm in all measurement planes. Macroadenomas, thus, are greater than 1 cm (**ii**). Small non-neoplastic pituitary cysts are also occasionally encountered but can often be distinguished from adenomas by their increased T2 signal.

PATHOLOGY AND CLINICAL CORRELATION Pituitary adenomas account for approximately 15% of intracranial neoplasms and can cause symptoms either by mass effect or endocrine imbalance (**iii**). Microadenomas are small by definition and generally produce symptoms, if at all, by altered hormone production. Each pituitary cell type can form an adenoma and symptoms differ accordingly. Prolactin-secreting tumours (prolactinomas) are most common and can cause amenorrhea, infertility, and galactorrhea. Other functioning adenoma subtypes secrete growth hormone, adrenocorticotrophic hormone (ACTH), thyroid-stimulating hormone, or gonadotropins (leutenizing hormone and/or follicle stimulating hormone). Nonfunctioning adenomas also exist but are usually silent early and present as macroadenomas with symptoms related to mass effect.

Treatment varies by symptom and cellular subtype. Incidental adenomas can be safely observed by interval MRI. Symptomatic prolactinomas are generally treated with a dopamine agonist, with normalization of prolactin levels in approximately 80% of cases. Trans-sphenoidal surgery is reserved for refractory prolactinomas but is the mainstay for all other cell types. Radiosurgery is controversial, but has been applied to residual tumour remnants.

TEACHING PEARLS
➤ *Pituitary microadenomas measure less than 1 cm by definition.*
➤ *These lesions are conspicuous on postcontrast images, due to their relative lack of enhancement.*
➤ *Trans-sphenoidal resection is the mainstay of therapy for all cell types except in some cases prolactinomas.*

REFERENCES (CASE 92)

Kreutzer J, Fahlbusch R (2004). Diagnosis and treatment of pituitary tumours. *Curr Opin Neurol* **17**:693–703.

Shimon I, Melmed S (1998). Management of pituitary tumours. *Ann Intern Med* **129**(6)\:472–83.

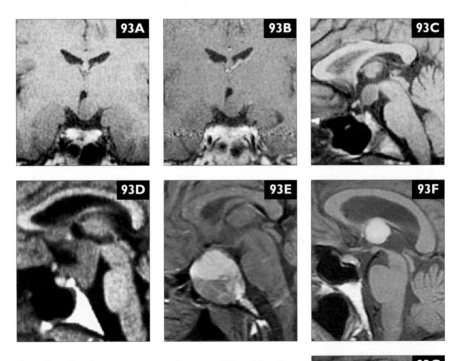

93 A female with precocious puberty and 'laughing fits' presents, and the following images are obtained (93A–C).

i. Where is the lesion located? Is it sellar or suprasellar?

ii. What is the differential diagnosis?

DIFFERENTIAL DIAGNOSIS Images 93D–G.

93 DIAGNOSIS Hypothalamic hamartoma.

IMAGING FINDINGS Images **93A–C** (coronal T1, coronal T1 post gadolinium, and sagittal T1, respectively) show a left-sided nonenhancing lesion in the substance of the hypothalamus. which is isointense to the grey matter. The lesion is suprasellar in location (**i**). The infundibulum, pituitary gland, and bony sella are normal in appearance.

DIFFERENTIAL DIAGNOSIS The differential diagnosis (**ii**) of a homogenous suprasellar mass includes:
- Chiasmatic glioma (see Question **94**).
- Hypothalamic glioma (**93D**, sagittal T1).
- Pituitary macroadenoma (**93E**, sagittal T1).
- Tuber cinereum hamartoma (**93A–C**).
- Meningioma.
- Colloid cyst (**93F**, sagittal T1).
- Dermoid (**93G**, sagittal T1).
- Lipoma.
- Plus differential diagnosis of heterogenous suprasellar mass (Question **96**).
- Plus differential diagnosis of pituitary stalk anomaly.

An accurate differential diagnosis relies on precise localization of the lesion: is it sellar, suprasellar, or both? Image **93D** shows a T1 isointense pilocytic astrocytoma originating from the hypothalamus. Contrast this suprasellar location with the lesion shown in **93E**, which reveals a large, round, well-defined macroadenoma that is both sellar and suprasellar in location; note that the macroadenoma obliterates the normal pituitary gland and remodels the bony sella. The internal signal characteristics suggest subacute internal haemorrhage, with an inferior T1 hypointense portion and a superior hyperintense portion. The colloid cyst in **93F** is attached to anterosuperior 3rd ventricular roof. The most common location of T1 hyperintense (typically fat-containing) dermoids is the suprasellar region (**93G**).

PATHOLOGY AND CLINICAL CORRELATION Hypothalamic hamartoma is a non-neoplastic congenital heterotopia of grey matter located in region of tuber cinereum. Patients are usually between 1 and 3 years old and typically present with luteinizing hormone releasing hormone (LHRH)-dependent central precocious puberty, including increased height and overweight with advanced bone age. Furthermore, patients suffer from gelastic (laughing/crying spells) seizures. Hormonal suppressive therapy with LHRH agonists is successful in most patients.

TEACHING PEARLS
> *In T1 and T2 hypothalamic hamartoma is isointense to grey matter, homogenous, nonenhancing, and a round tuber cinereum mass.*
> *Think of hamartoma in an infant with precocious puberty.*
> *Peak age is between 1 and 3 years old.*

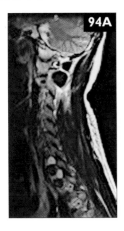

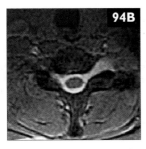

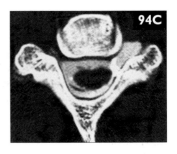

94 A 28-year-old male was involved in a motorcycle accident. He suffered left shoulder pain and arm weakness. The following images are obtained (**94A–C**).
i. What is the composition of the abnormal neural foramen?
ii. What might it indicate?

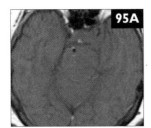

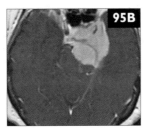

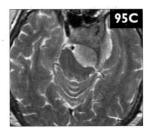

95 A companion case to Question 91 (chondrosarcoma) presents, and the following images are obtained (**95A–C**).
i. Where is the lesion located?
ii. What imaging sequences were used and what are the imaging characteristics of the lesion?

94 DIAGNOSIS Nerve root avulsions.

IMAGING FINDINGS T2-weighted imaging reveals ovoid areas of CSF signal intensity (**i**) extending through the left neural foramena of C7/T1 and T1/T2 levels. Findings are in keeping with pseudomeningoceles from nerve root avulsion (**ii**). CT myelography confirms the finding.

DIFFERENTIAL DIAGNOSIS A lateral thoracic meningocoele, most commonly found in neurofibromatosis, may have similar imaging findings. A neurofibroma should also be considered when a mass is found in the neural foramen – unlike a nerve root avulsion, this should enhance.

PATHOLOGY AND CLINICAL CORRELATION The diagnosis is best confirmed on imaging by MRI or CT myelography. Imaging should ideally differentiate between a pre- and post-ganglionic injury as only the latter are amenable to repair. Images should be evaluated for the presence of intradural nerve roots or a root stump, deformities of the nerve sleeve, as well as the presence of a meningocoele.

TEACHING PEARL
➤ *A nerve root avulsion should be suspected when a pseudomeningocoele in seen in a neural foramen, post trauma.*

REFERENCE
Volle E, *et al.* (1992). Radicular avulsion resulting from spinal injury: assessment of diagnostic modalities. *Neuroradiology* 34:235–40.

95 DIAGNOSIS Meningioma.

IMAGING FINDINGS Images **95A–C** show a T1 isointense, homogenously enhancing meningioma in the region of the left cavernous sinus, with mass effect on the left cerebral peduncle and involvement of the left chiasm and optic nerve. Encasement and displacement of the basilar artery is noted, without narrowing. There is also enhancement of the left tentorium cerebelli (**i, ii**).

DIFFERENTIAL DIAGNOSIS See Question **91** for a full discussion of the differential diagnosis.

TEACHING PEARLS
➤ *Meningioma is an extra-axial sharply circumscribed smooth parasellar mass abutting dura, sometimes with a dural tail.*
➤ *There is homogenous and intense enhancement.*
➤ *There is hyperostosis, irregular cortex, and calcifications.*
➤ *Most common meningioma locations include: parasagittal/convexity (50%), sphenoid ridge (20%), parasellar (10%), cerebellopontine angle (10%), olfactory groove (5%).*

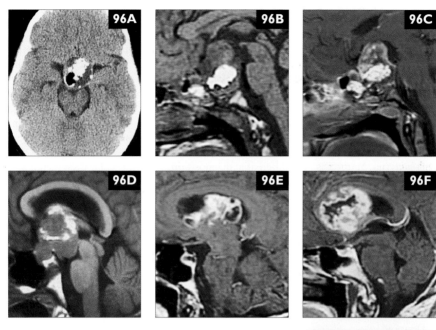

96 A 9-year-old girl presents with morning headache, and the following images are obtained (96A–C).

i. What is the morphology and enhancement pattern of the lesion?

ii. What structures of the brain are affected?

iii. What is the differential diagnosis in this region?

DIFFERENTIAL DIAGNOSIS Images 96D–G.

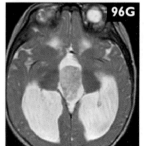

96 DIAGNOSIS Craniopharyngioma (CP).

IMAGING FINDINGS Images **96A–C** (axial unenhanced CT, sagittal T1, sagittal contrast-enhanced T1, respectively) demonstrate a complex, partially cystic, strongly calcified suprasellar mass. The solid portions enhance heterogeneously, and there is intrinsic T1 hyperintensity within the mass, which most likely reflects high protein content (**i**). There is an ovoid hypodensity within the mass (representing either air or fat). The tumour fills the 3rd ventricle, causing cranial deviation of the fornix and interthalamic adhesion and effacement of the lateral ventricle (**ii**).

DIFFERENTIAL DIAGNOSIS The differential diagnosis (**iii**) of a suprasellar mass includes:
In children:
- CP (**96A–C**).
- Glioma (e.g. pilocytic astrocytoma) (see Question **100**).
- Germinoma (**96D**, sagittal T1).
- Hypothalamic hamartoma.
- Supratentorial primitive neuroectodermal tumour (PNET) (**96E**, sagittal contrast-enhanced T1).
- Atypical teratoid-rhabdoid tumour (**96G**, axial T2).
- Embryonal carcinoma.
- Teratoma.
- Dermoid.
In adults:
- Macroadenoma.
- Meningioma.
- Glioma.
- Craniopharyngioma.
- Aneurysm.
- Metastases.
- Glioblastoma multiforme (GBM) (**96F**, sagittal contrast-enhanced T1).

An accurate differential diagnosis relies on precise localization of the lesion: is it sellar, suprasellar, or both? The germinoma in **96D**, with prominent posterior extension and patchy T1 hyperintense haemorrhage resembles CP. In contrast to CP, germinomas are typically noncystic and noncalcified. Supratentorial PNETs (**96E**) are typically heterogenous like CPs due to haemorrhage and calcifications, but are rarely seen in the supratentorial region. Image **96F** depicts a GBM arising from the corpus callosum and extending into the lateral and 3rd ventricle. Although more often seen infratentorial, atypical teratoid-rhabdoid tumours (**96G**) also affect the suprasellar region and should be considered in male children under age 3 years.

PATHOLOGY AND CLINICAL CORRELATION CPs are slow growing WHO grade 1 tumours arising from metaplasia of squamous epithelial remnants (Rathke pouch) of the adenohypophysis. About 50% of all paediatric sellar/suprasellar region tumours are CPs. They present in a bimodal age distribution with one peak in children between 5 and 15 years and the other peak in adults older than 50 years. The more cystic, calcified, and recurrent adamantinomatous type of CP occurs more often in the younger, while the more solid-appearing papillary type can be seen in an older age group. Although symptoms vary with location, size of tumour and age of patient, the typical clinical presentation is a paediatric patient with morning headache, visual defect, and short stature.

TEACHING PEARLS
➤ *CP is the most common sellar/suprasellar region mass in a child.*
➤ *Rarely, lesions can be purely sellar at presentation.*
➤ *CPs are multiplilobulated, multicystic, in 90% calcified heterogeneously enhancing suprasellar masses.*
➤ *It is a benign, slow growing tumour with 75% overall 10-year survival.*
➤ *There are two age peaks: 5–15 years and >50-year-old patients.*

REFERENCES
Van Effenterre R, Boch AL (2002). Craniopharyngioma in adults and children: a study of 122 surgical cases. *J Neurosurg* 97(1):3–11.
Osborn AG, *et al.* (2004). *Brain.* Amirsys, Salt Lake City, Chapter I-6, pp. 30–33.

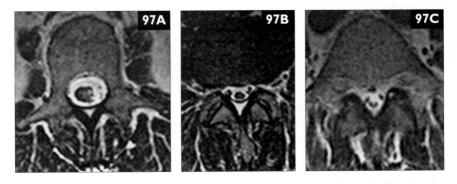

97 A patient presents with severe back pain following surgery 8 months previously. The following images are obtained (**97A–C**).
i. What is the primary finding in these axial images through the cauda equina?
ii. Is this process amenable to surgical therapy?

97 **DIAGNOSIS** Arachnoiditis.

IMAGING FINDINGS These three axial T2 images (**97A–C**) are all through the cauda equina inferior to the termination of the spinal cord. Extensive nerve root clumping is seen (**i**). This finding is most pronounced in image **97A** where nearly all of the roots are clumped together to the right of midline simulating a solid mass. No enhancement was seen following contrast administration.

DIFFERENTIAL DIAGNOSIS Clumped nerve roots suggest arachnoiditis. This is especially true in the postoperative patient. Possible mimics include tumours of the nerve root sheaths or intrathecal metastases, both of which should enhance.

PATHOLOGY AND CLINICAL CORRELATION Arachnoiditis is an intrathecal inflammatory reaction most commonly seen following lumbar spinal surgery. Historically, this process was associated with myelographic contrast dye exposure but modern, nonionic water-soluble agents have made this much less common. Patients can present with varied symptoms. Pain is usually severe and can be localized or radiating. Paraparesis, gait disorders, and bladder or bowel dysfunction can also be seen. It is not uncommon for patients with active arachnoiditis to have severe pain with lumbar puncture (which can aid in diagnosis). Interestingly, imaging findings do not appear to correlate with symptoms.

Arachnoiditis is manifest radiographically by nerve root adhesion. Roots can adhere to each other, as in this case, or can adhere to the dura causing an 'empty thecal sac' sign. In severe cases, adhesions can compartmentalize the thecal sac causing unusual filling during myelography.

Treatment is by intrathecal administration of steroids or by spinal cord stimulation. Surgical treatment is generally avoided as this usually makes the inflammation worse (**ii**).

TEACHING PEARLS
➤ *Arachnoiditis can manifest as nerve root clumping or the 'empty thecal sac' sign (roots adherent to the thecal sac peripherally).*
➤ *Arachnoiditis is a cause of 'failed back syndrome' following lumbar surgery.*

REFERENCES
Ross JS (2000). Magnetic resonance imaging of the postoperative spine. *Semin Musculoskelet Radiol* 4(3):281–91.
Ross JS, *et al.* (1987). MR imaging of lumbar arachnoiditis. *AJR* 149:1025–32.
Smith AS, Blaser SI (1991). Infectious and inflammatory processes of the spine. *Radiol Clin North Am* 29(4):809–27.
Teplick JG, Haskin ME (1983). Computed tomography of the postoperative lumbar spine. *AJR* 141(5):865–84.

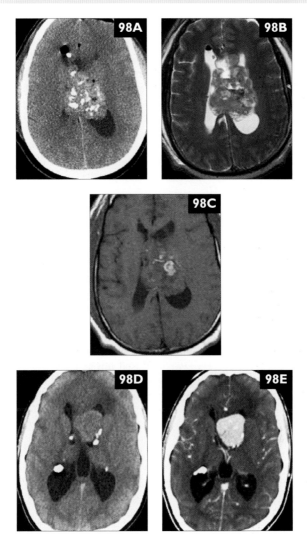

98 A 31-year-old male presents with headache and mental status change. The following images are obtained (98A–C).

i. Where is the mass located?

ii. Describe the morphology and signal characteristics of the tumour.

iii. What complication is seen?

iv. What is the differential diagnosis of a lesion in this location?

DIFFERENTIAL DIAGNOSIS Images 98D, E.

98 **DIAGNOSIS** Central neurocytoma.

IMAGING FINDINGS Images 98A–C (axial NECT, axial T2, axial T1, respectively) demonstrate a circumscribed, lobulated heterogenous mass localized in the body of the lateral ventricle crossing midline (i). Multiple calcifications are seen in NECT and intratumoral cysts are visible in the T2-weighted scan (ii). Hydrocephalus secondary to foramen of Monro obstruction is associated with the mass (iii). Note also the intraventricular and extra-axial gas, reflecting recent biopsy.

DIFFERENTIAL DIAGNOSIS The differential diagnosis (iv) of masses located in the lateral ventricle or along the margin of the lateral ventricle include:
• Central neurocytoma (98A–C).
• Subependymoma (see Question 89).
• Subependmyal giant cell astrocytoma (98D, E, axial unenhanced CT, axial contrast enhanced CT).
• Plus: differential diagnosis of trigonal lateral ventricle mass (see Question 102).
Images 98D, E demonstrates multiple calcified subependymal nodules in the body and atrium of the lateral ventricle bilaterally. A large noncalcified intensely enhancing mass in the left frontal horn near the foramen of Monro displaces the septum pellucidum to the right and is consistent with a subependymal giant cell astrocytoma.

PATHOLOGY AND CLINICAL CORRELATION Neurocytoma is an intraventricular WHO grade 2 neuroepithelial tumour with neuronal differentiation. Patients typically present with headache, seizures and/or increased intracranial pressure secondary to hydrocephalus due to foramen of Monro obstruction. After complete surgical resection as primary treatment of this benign tumour, local recurrence is rare and 5-year survival is about 85%.

TEACHING PEARLS
➤ *Consider central neurocytoma in a multilobulated, often calcified, heterogeneously enhancing mass in a young adult.*
➤ *It is usually attached to the septum pellucidum.*
➤ *Age peak is 20–40 years; mean patient age is 30 years.*

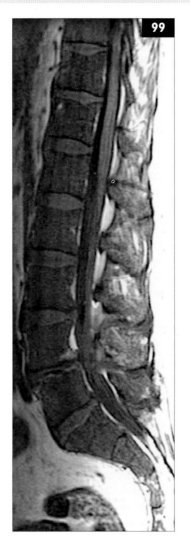

99 A 50-year-old male patient with anaemia and back pain underwent an MRI (**99**).
i. What sequence is this?
ii. What abnormality is shown?

99 DIAGNOSIS Diffuse marrow replacement.

IMAGING FINDINGS On a T1-weighted image in an adult, the fatty marrow should be brighter than the intervertebral discs. In this pathologic case, marrow is diffusely dark on T1-weighted imaging (i, ii).

DIFFERENTIAL DIAGNOSIS Marrow reconversion (see below) can be seen as a normal finding in heavy smokers. More patchy marrow changes may be seen in degenerative change, malignancy, and infection.

PATHOLOGY AND CLINICAL CORRELATION In childhood, bone marrow is a site of active haematopoiesis. By adulthood, however, bone marrow converts into inactive marrow, with a much higher fat composition and subsequently appears bright on T1-weighted imaging. Marrow can be 'reconverted' into active marrow in adults should increased haematopoiesis be required, e.g. anaemia, and marrow replacement disorders, e.g. myelofibrosis.

TEACHING PEARL
➤ *Spinal bone marrow should be brighter than intervertebral discs in adults on T1-weighted imaging.*

REFERENCE
Poulton TB, *et al*. (1993). Bone marrow reconversion in adults who are smokers: MR imaging findings. *AJR* **161**(6):1217–21.

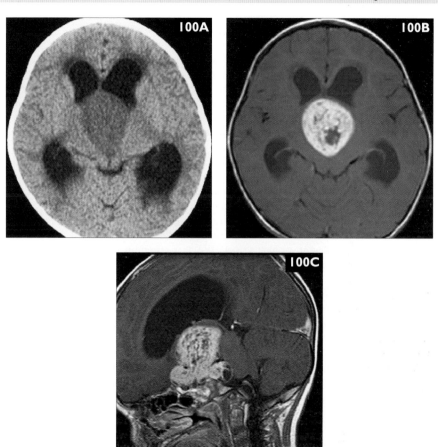

100 An 8-year-old female presents with vision changes, and the following images are obtained (**100A–C**).
i. What is the morphology and enhancement pattern of the lesion?
ii. What structures of the brain are affected?

100 DIAGNOSIS Optic chiasm glioma (juvenile pilocytic astrocytoma).

IMAGING FINDINGS Images **100A–C** demonstrate a CT hypodense, round, well demarcated, strongly enhancing juvenile pilocytic astrocytoma (JPA) with nonspecific T1 hypointense nonenhancing foci, possibly representing small cysts or necrotic areas (**i**). The mass expands the 3rd ventricle blocking the foramen of Monro, causing marked hydrocephalus, and is sufficiently large such that the region of origin – either the hypothalamus or the optic chiasm – is uncertain (**ii**).

DIFFERENTIAL DIAGNOSIS The differential diagnosis of a suprasellar mass in a child includes craniopharyngioma, optic nerve glioma, germinoma, hypothalamic hamartoma, supratentorial primitive neuroectodermal tumour (PNET), atypical teratoid–rhaboid tumour, embryonal carcinoma, teratoma, and dermoid. The precise differential diagnosis is dependent on localizing the lesion as sellar, suprasellar, or both.

PATHOLOGY AND CLINICAL CORRELATION JPA is a common intracranial tumour of childhood. Lesions occur in one of two characteristic locations: the cerebellum or the optic pathway (optic nerve, optic chiasm, or optic tract). Optic tract lesions result in enlargement of the involved structures. There is a close relationship between optic nerve JPAs and neurofibromatosis type 1: 33% of patients with this entity have NF1 and 15% of patients with NF1 will develop a pilocytic astrocytoma.

TEACHING PEARLS
- *Pilocytic astrocytoma: most common primary brain tumour in children; typically a cystic appearing cerebellar lesion with enhancing mural nodule lateral to the 4th ventricle (primary differential diagnosis is hemangioblastoma, a more rare lesion associated with Von Hippel–Lindau syndrome).*
- *Lesions can appear aggressive but are easily treated.*
- *Remember the association between chiasmatic JPA and neurofibromatosis 1: up to 1/3 of patients with optic pathway JPAs have NF1.*
- *Mean patient age: 5-15 years.*

REFERENCES
Bernaerts A, *et al.* (2003). Juvenile pilocytic astrocytoma. *JBR-BTR* **86**(3):142–3.
Osborn AG, *et al.* (2004). *Brain*. Amirsys, Salt Lake City, Chapter I-6, pp. 30–3.

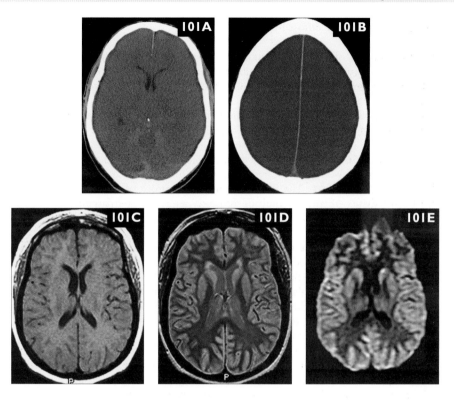

101 A 14-year-old child is admitted following near-drowning. The following images are obtained (**101A, B**).

i. Is symmetry on CT a reliable indicator of normalcy?

ii. What is the most sensitive region of the brain to hypoxia?

COMPANION CASE

A 57-year-old presents following cardiac arrest, and the following images are obtained (**101C–E**).

101 DIAGNOSIS Severe diffuse hypoxic injury.

IMAGING FINDINGS There is complete loss of grey–white matter differentiation on CT (**101A, B**). Diffuse symmetric cerebral oedema is manifest by loss of sulcal margins. The falx cerebri and tentorium appear relatively bright compared to the diffuse hypoattenuation of the adjacent brain.

The companion case demonstrates subtle diffuse cortical and basal ganglia T1 hypointensity (**101C**) and intermediate/T2 hyperintensity (**101D**). The diffusion-weighted image (**101E**) displays increased signal corresponding to restricted diffusion throughout the cortical and deep grey nuclei.

DIFFERENTIAL DIAGNOSIS The findings are manifestations of diffuse anoxic injury. Common causes of anoxia include hypoglycemia; near drowning; hanging; hypotension; as well as carbon monoxide, cyanide, or methanol poisoning.

PATHOLOGY AND CLINICAL CORRELATION Anoxia leads to cellular infarction and associated cytotoxic oedema. There are a variety of imaging findings in diffuse hypoxia along a spectrum related to the degree of oxygen deprivation. In radiology, symmetry is often a useful feature in evaluating for pathology. Unfortunately, this is usually not the case when assessing for diffuse hypoxia (**i**). Findings may be seen in the basal ganglia (the most sensitive region to anoxic injury) (**ii**), within the border zones between vascular distributions, or globally (as in this case). Generally, grey matter is more sensitive to hypoxia than white matter. As CT is often used as an initial imaging modality, it is important to be familiar with the CT appearance of this devastating process. Once the diagnosis is suggested, MRI imaging should be performed for confirmation. Diffusion-weighted imaging is a sensitive and specific means to evaluate for ischaemia in adults, but may be less sensitive in the neonatal period. As the companion case demonstrates, symmetric areas of diffusion restriction can also be difficult to recognize.

TEACHING PEARLS
- ➤ *Diffuse cerebral hypoxia manifests as symmetric hypoattenuation, loss of grey–white differentiation, and oedema on CT imaging.*
- ➤ *Findings can be seen focally in the basal ganglia or border zones, or diffusely throughout the brain.*

REFERENCES
Forbes KPN, Pipe JG, Bird R (2000). Neonatal hypoxic-ischaemic encephalopathy: detection with diffusion-weighted MR imaging. *AJNR* 21:1490–6.

Han BK, *et al.* (1989). Reversal sign on CT: effect of anoxic/ischaemic cerebral injury in children. *AJNR* 10:1191–8.

Kjos BO, Brant-Zawadzki M, Young RG (1983). Early CT findings of global central nervous system hypoperfusion. *AJR* 141:1227–32.

Ohkawa S, Yamadori A (1993). CT in hanging. *Neuroradiology* 35:591.

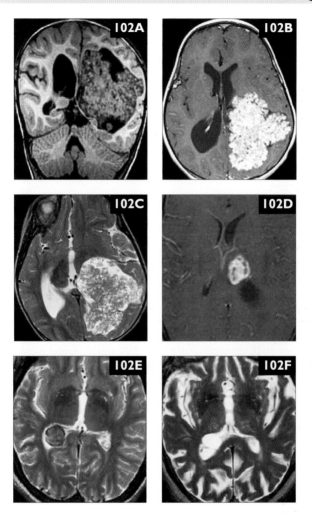

102 A 6-month-old boy presents with a head circumference above the 99th percentile. The following images are obtained (102A–C).

i. Where is the mass located?

ii. Describe the morphology, signal characterics, and enhancement pattern of the lesion.

iii. What is the differential diagnosis in this region of the brain?

DIFFERENTIAL DIAGNOSIS Images 102D–F.

102 DIAGNOSIS Choroid plexus papilloma (CPP).

IMAGING FINDINGS Images **102A–C** (coronal T1, axial contrast-enhanced T1, axial T2, respectively) show a T1 isointense, T2 hyperintense, strongly enhancing lobulated mass with a frond-like surface in the trigone of the left lateral ventricle. Cerebrospinal fluid (CSF) is trapped between the papillae, giving the lesion a mottled appearance on T1 and T2 (**i,ii**). Ventricular enlargement is consistent with hydrocephalus.

DIFFERENTIAL DIAGNOSIS The differential diagnosis (**iii**) of a trigonal lateral ventricle mass includes:
Characteristic frond-like appearance:
• CPP (**102A–C**).
• Choroid plexus carcinoma (see Question **109**).
Other trigonal masses:
• Ependymoma
• Choroidal metastasis (**102D**, axial contrast-enhanced T1).
• Trigonal meningioma (**102E**, axial T2).
• Choroid plexus cyst (**102F**, axial T2).
The differential diagnosis of lesions in the trigones of the lateral ventricles is highly dependent on age. Choroid plexus papilloma and carcinoma cannot be differentiated with imaging alone, although very aggressive features might suggest the latter diagnosis. Image **102D** shows a strongly enhancing renal cell carcinoma metastasis in a 63-year-old patient. Image **102E** demonstrates a well demarcated, round meningioma in a 41-year-old, and **102F** depicts multiple T2 hyperintense choroid plexus cysts.

PATHOLOGY AND CLINICAL CORRELATION CPP is a intraventricular papillary neoplasm derived from the choroid plexus epithelium. The most frequent locations are the atrium of the lateral ventricle and the 4th ventricle. CPP is the most common tumour in children under age 1 year, and presents with macrocephaly and bulging fontanelle secondary to hydrocephalus. Diffuse hydrocephalus is either due to CSF overproduction, mechanical obstruction, or impaired CSF resorption because of haemorrhage. CSF dissemination is possible, mandating screening of the entire spine for drop metastasis.

TEACHING PEARLS
➤ *CPP is a strongly enhancing intraventricular frond-like mass.*
➤ *It is the most common brain tumour in children <1 year.*
➤ *It presents with macrocephaly and bulging fontanelle due to hydrocephalus.*
➤ *Perform contrast-enhanced MR of entire neuraxis before surgery.*
➤ *One cannot differentiate between choroid plexus papillomas and carcinomas on the basis of imaging alone.*

REFERENCES
Knierim DS, *et al.* (1991). Choroid plexus tumour in infants. *Pediatr Neurosurg* **16**: 276–80.
Osborn AG, *et al.* (2004). *Brain.* Amirsys, Salt Lake City, Chapter I-6, pp. 60–65.

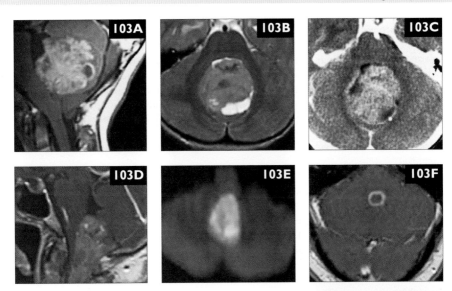

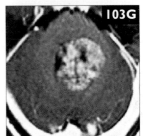

103 A 3-year-old boy presents with ataxia and vomiting. The following images are obtained (103A–C).

i. Where is the lesion located?

ii. What other MR studies would you request and what would you look for?

iii. What is the differential diagnosis for this mass?

DIFFERENTIAL DIAGNOSIS Images 103D–G.

103 DIAGNOSIS Medulloblastoma.

IMAGING FINDINGS Images **103A–C** (sagittal contrast-enhanced T1, axial T2, axial contrast-enhanced CT, respectively) demonstrate a heterogeneously enhancing well demarcated papillary mass expanding the 4th ventricle and elevating the superior medullary velum (**i**). The hyperintense foci within the mass on T2-weighted images are due to small cysts, while the hypointense foci are due to calcifications.

DIFFERENTIAL DIAGNOSIS The differential diagnosis (**iii**) of a 4th ventricle mass includes:
• Medulloblastoma (**103A-C**).
• Ependymoma (see Question **108**).
• Pilocytic astrocytoma.
• Subependymoma (**103D**, sagittal contrast-enhanced T1).
• Epidermoid (**103E**, axial DWI).
• Metastasis (**103F**, axial contrast-enhanced T1).
• Atypical teratoid-rhabdoid tumour (**103G**, axial contrast-enhanced T1).
Location can help determine the tumour type (see Teaching pearls). Patient age is also crucial in differentiating different 4th ventricular tumours. Subependymomas (**103D**) typically occur in middle-aged or elderly patients. Metastases (**103F**) are often multiple, occurring generally in older patients. Epidermoids (**103E**) show restricted diffusion in the DWI sequence. Atypical teratoid-rhabdoid tumours (**103G**) are more heterogenous than medulloblastomas due to cysts, haemorrhage, or calcifications and children are typically under 3 years old.

PATHOLOGY AND CLINICAL CORRELATION Medulloblastoma is a malignant, invasive, highly cellular embryonal tumour, classified as grade 4 by the WHO and typically arising from the roof of the 4th ventricle. Medulloblastomas represent 15–20% of all paediatric brain tumours. They are diagnosed mostly by age 5 years in children, presenting with ataxia and vomiting due to local mass effect and/or increased intracranial pressure secondary to hydrocephalus. Medulloblastomas are fast growing and about 20% of cases demonstrate cerebrospinal fluid (CSF) dissemination at the time of diagnosis. For this reason, a directed search for CSF dissemination is necessary for treatment planning, with imaging evaluation of the entire neuraxis (**ii**). This initial screen and the postoperative evaluation of surgical bed are key to prognosis, which varies between 20 and 100% 5-year survival rate. Treatment is surgical excision with adjuvant radiation and chemotherapy.

TEACHING PEARLS

➤ *Medulloblastoma is the second most common posterior fossa tumour in children (after juvenile pilocytic astrocytoma, JPA).*

➤ *It is a heterogenous, solid, enhancing WHO grade 4 tumour, originating at the roof of the 4th ventricle.*

➤ *The location relative to the 4th ventricle is crucial: if anterior in the brainstem consider glioma or demyelination; within and extending via foramen of Luschka consider ependymoma; posterior along the posterior margin of the ventricle consider medulloblastoma/ primitive neuroectodermal tumour, and lateral in the cerebellar hemispheres consider JPA.*

➤ *Enhancing mural nodules should raise the differential of JPA, von Hippel-Lindau (look for renal or spinal manifestations), or haemangioblastoma (in an older patient).*

➤ *Contrast-enhanced MR of the entire neuraxis is essential to detect CSF dissemination.*

REFERENCE

Koeller KK, Rushing EJ (2003). Medulloblastoma: a comprehensive review with radiologic-pathologic correlation. *Radiographics* **23**:1613–37.

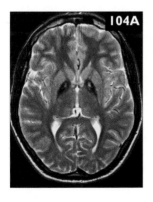 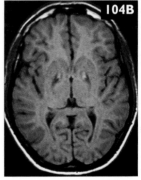

104 A patient presents with speech disturbance, and the following images are obtained (**104A, B**).

i. What structure is abnormal?

ii. What is the name given to this classic imaging appearance?

iii. What syndrome is most commonly associated with this sign?

104 **DIAGNOSIS** Hallervorden–Spatz syndrome (HS).

IMAGING FINDINGS There is marked signal hypointensity on this T2-weighted image (**104A**) circumpherentially surrounding a central region of high signal intensity in the anteromedial globus pallidi (**i**). The T1-weighted image (**104B**) shows similar, though less pronounced findings. This appearance constitutes the classic 'eye-of-the-tiger' sign (**ii**).

DIFFERENTIAL DIAGNOSIS The 'eye-of-the-tiger'sign is closely associated with HS, but can also be seen with other rare extrapyramidal parkinsonian disorders including cortical-basal ganglionic degeneration, early onset levodopa-unresponsive parkinsonism, and progressive supranuclear palsy (**iii**). Other entities involving the basal ganglia are cyanide or carbon monoxide poisoning, Wilson's disease, Leigh's disease, hypoxemia, and hypotension.

PATHOLOGY AND CLINICAL CORRELATION HS or pantothenate kinase-associated neurodegeneration (PKAN), is a progressive neurodegenerative disorder characterized by extrapyramidal and pyramidal signs, dystonia, dysarthria, and iron accumulation in the globus pallidi and brainstem nuclei. The pathophysiologic basis of excess iron accumulation and toxicity is currently hypothetical but an increased level of cysteine (due to enzymatic deficiency) may serve as a chelating agent. Interestingly, blood and CSF iron levels remain normal.

HS has two distinct forms clinically. Classic disease shows early onset and rapid progression. The atypical form is characterized by later onset (in the teen years) and a slower progression. Cases are evenly divided between sporadic and familial forms (through autosomal recessive inheritance). Prior to MRI, the diagnosis was only confirmed at autopsy. The disease progresses to death, early in the classic form and later with the atypical variant. No cure exists.

TEACHING PEARLS
➤ *The 'eye-of-the-tiger' sign suggests HS.*
➤ *HS is due to excess iron accumulation in the globus pallidi.*

REFERENCES
Guillerman RP (2000). The eye-of-the-tiger sign. *Radiology* **217**:895–6.
Hayflick SJ, *et al.* (2003). Genetic, clinical, and radiographic delineation of Hallervorden–Spatz syndrome. *N Eng J Med* **348**(1):33–40.
Sener RN (2003). Pantothenate kinase-associated neurodegeneration: MR imaging, proton MR spectroscopy, and diffusion MR imaging findings. *AJNR* **24**:1690–3.

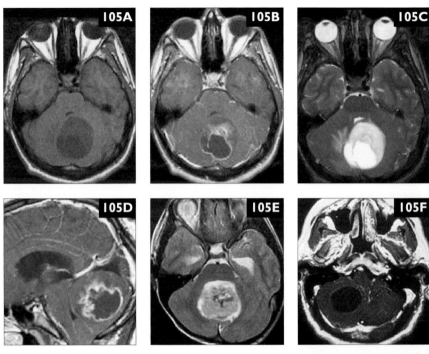

105 A 15-year-old boy presents with ataxia and headache. The following images are obtained (105A–D).

i. Where is the mass located and what is its relation to the 4th ventricle?

ii. What are the components of the mass?

iii. What is the differential diagnosis?

DIFFERENTIAL DIAGNOSIS Images 105E–G.

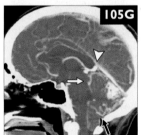

203

105 **Diagnosis** Juvenile pilocytic astrocytoma (JPA).

Imaging findings Images 105A–D (axial T1, axial contrast-enhanced T1, axial T2, sagittal contrast-enhanced T1, respectively) demonstrate a mildly enhancing cerebellar mass with a large cystic component (ii). Enhancement is heterogenous and includes wall of cyst. The tumour is located within the left cerebellar hemisphere, causing diplacement and effacement of the 4th ventricle (i).

Differential diagnosis The differential diagnosis (iii) of a cerebellar mass includes:
In children:
• Pilocytic astrocytoma (105A–D).
• Medulloblastoma/ primitive neuroectodermal tumour (105E, axial T2).
• Ependymoma.
In adults:
• Metastasis (105F, axial contrast-enhanced T1).
• Haemangioblastoma (see Question 111).
• Astrocytoma.
• Arteriovenous malformation (105G, axial contrast-enhanced T1).
In children, the key to the differential diagnosis of posterior fossa lesions is position relative to the 4th ventricle. Brainstem gliomas and demyelination occur anterior to the 4th ventricle, JPAs are posterolateral in the cerebellar hemispheres, medulloblastomas are located at the roof of the 4th ventricle, and ependymomas grow out of the 4th ventricle via the foramina.

The rim-enhancing cyst in image 105F represents a metastasis from angiosarcoma of the masticator space; the lesion is indistinguishable from a JPA or haemangioblastoma. The arteriovenous malformation in image 105G can be diagnosed by noting the enlarged superior cerebellar artery (white arrow) and posterior inferior cerebellar artery (black arrow) as feeding vessels and an enlarged vein of Galen and straight sinus (white arrowhead) as draining veins.

Pathology and clinical correlation JPA is a well-circumscribed, often cystic, slow growing WHO grade 1 tumour. The cerebellum is affected in 60% and the optic nerve in 30% of cases. Cerebellar JPA is the most common posterior fossa neoplasm in the paediatric age group and is typically characterized by a large cystic component with an enhancing mural nodule. Patients are children who present with headache and vomiting as a consequence of hydrocephalus due to compression of the 4th ventricle.

Teaching pearls
➤ *JPA is the most common posterior fossa tumour in children.*
➤ *It is a cystic cerebellar mass with enhancing solid nodule.*
➤ *Origin from the hemispheres and compression of the 4th ventricle typically distinguishes JPA from medulloblastoma, which expands the 4th ventricle after arising from its roof.*
➤ *Age peak is 5–15 years.*

REFERENCE (CASE 105)
Bernaerts A, *et al.* (2003). Juvenile pilocytic astrocytoma. *JBR-BTR* 86(3):142–3.

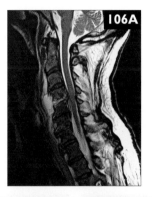

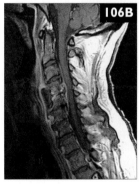

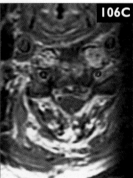

106 A 78-year-old diabetic patient presents with severe neck pain. The following images are obtained (**106A–C**).
i. What disc space level is abnormal?
ii. What is the specific space within the osseous spinal canal showing abnormal enhancement (**106B, C**)?
iii. What is the treatment for this process?

106 DIAGNOSIS Epidural abscess complicating cervical discitis.

IMAGING FINDINGS The sagittal T2-weighted image (**106A**) demonstrates hyperintense signal within the C4–5 disk space and a sizable prevertebral fluid collection (**i**). Osseous endplate irregularities are noted at the adjacent vertebral endplates. After gadolinium administration, the sagittal T1 image demonstrates enhancement within the disc space as well as circumferentially around the prevertebral collection (**106B**). In addition, there is enhancing soft tissue within the ventral epidural space posterior to both the C4 and C5 vertebral bodies (**ii**). The axial postcontrast T1 image (**106C**) confirms the epidural enhancement and demonstrates narrowing of the spinal canal and mild contouring of the left ventral cord. Cord signal is normal.

DIFFERENTIAL DIAGNOSIS The findings are extremely worrisome for focal discitis and associated prevertebral and epidural abscess. However, differential considerations could include sterile haematoma (in the setting of trauma), discitis alone, and possibly postoperative granulation tissue.

PATHOLOGY AND CLINICAL CORRELATION This case demonstrates the classic appearance of an epidural abscess. These infections are usually caused by local spread from discitis or other infection in the region. Less commonly, the epidural space is infected by haematogenous dissemination, open trauma, or recent surgery. As is often the case, it is the elderly or immunocompromised patient who is most at risk of developing an abscess. The infectious agent is most commonly *Staphylococcus aureus*, followed by *Mycobacterium tuberculosis*. The term 'abscess' is used slightly more loosely in the epidural space than in most other regions of the body. In general, any focal infection within the epidural space (whether loosely organized phlegmon or classic encapsulated fluid collection) is termed an abscess.

Imaging findings are those of discitis when present. Abscesses generally show fluid intensity (hypo/insointense T1, hyperintense T2/STIR) and enhance either diffusely or peripherally along the fluid margin. Pre- or paravertebral soft tissue abscesses are often present. Careful evaluation for spinal cord compression is imperative as symptoms of compression can be masked by the generally poor status of many patients. Abnormal signal within the cord suggests cord compression, ischaemia, or direct infection.

Treatment is usually surgical decompression and evacuation (performed on an emergent basis) with concurrent and long-term antibiotic coverage (**iii**). The development of an epidural abscess is an ominous occurrence as mortality reaches 1/3 of patients involved.

TEACHING PEARLS
➤ *Epidural enhancement associated with discitis or a paravertebral fluid collection is worrisome for abscess.*
➤ *Treatment is emergent surgical decompression and evacuation.*

REFERENCES (CASE 106)
Reihsaus E, Waldbaur H, Seeling W (2000). Spinal epidural abscess: a meta-analysis
  of 915 patients. *Neurosurg Rev* **23**(4):175–205.
Tung GA, *et al.* (1999). Spinal epidural abscess: correlation between MRI findings
  and outcome. *Neuroradiology* **41**(12):904–9.
Varma R, Lander P, Assaf A (2001). Imaging of pyogenic infectious spondylodiskitis.
  Radiol Clin N Am **39**(2):203–13.

107 A patient presents with bi-temporal hemi-anopsia and the following images are obtained (107A–C).

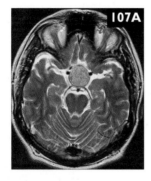

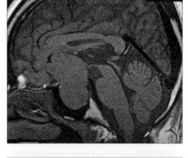

i. Do patients with large pituitary lesions generally present with endocrine symptoms?

ii. Which cell type is most common in these tumours?

iii. What structure is being superiorly displaced by the suprasellar component of this mass?

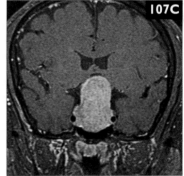

107 DIAGNOSIS Pitui-
tary macroadenoma.

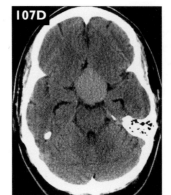

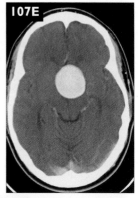

IMAGING FINDINGS

There is a 2.8 × 2.8 ×
4.7 cm mass within the
sella turcica and supra-
sellar region that shows
heterogeneous signal
intensity on axial T2
(**107A**). The T1 signal is
isointense to brain on
sagittal (**107B**) images.
This mass diffusely

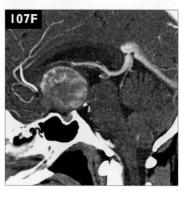

enhances and is shown to cause mass effect
upon the overlying optic chiasm on coronal
postcontrast T1 imaging (**107C**) (**iii**). The mass
abuts the medial wall of the cavernous sinus,
though clear sinus invasion is not seen. Normal
cavernous carotid artery flow voids are seen
bilaterally.

The companion case images (**107D–F**)
demonstrate another large suprasellar mass.
This lesion is hyperdense on noncontrast CT
and shows marked homogeneous enhancement
following contrast administration (**107D, E**).
Sagittal image from a CT arteriogram (**107F**)
gives the impression of swirling blood/contrast in this large anterior communicating
artery aneurysm.

DIFFERENTIAL DIAGNOSIS Suprasellar masses are commonly seen and the standard
differential can be recalled by the aid of a popular mnemonic 'SATCHMO'
(suprasellar extent of pituitary adenoma/sarcoid, aneurysm, teratoma [or other germ
cell tumour], craniopharyngioma, hypothalamic glioma or hamartoma,
meningioma/mets, and optic glioma/other). In this case, the sella appears widened
suggesting that the mass arises from the pituitary itself. Adenomas comprise the large
majority of pituitary masses though gland hyperplasia, lymphocytic hypophysitis, and
glandular haemorrhage should also be considered (**ii**). By definition, a pituitary
adenoma greater than 1 cm in size is termed a macroadenoma.

The companion case is also a suprasellar mass. The intense enhancement suggests the
correct diagnosis of giant aneurysm, confirmed by CT angiography (CTA). This case
should be a reminder that aneurysm is clearly in the differential for suprasellar lesions and
should be considered in all cases. Obviously, a biopsy of this lesion would be disastrous.

PATHOLOGY AND CLINICAL CORRELATION Pituitary macroadenomas can show endocrine function but are usually less active than microadenomas and, therefore, come to medical attention later in the disease process (**i**). Clinical symptoms generally relate to mass effect upon adjacent structures. The classic symptom is that of bilateral temporal visual field defects due to central mass effect upon the overlying optic chiasm. Lateral invasion into the cavernous sinuses can also become symptomatic with a variety of cranial nerve defects. These tumours are benign and usually grow very slowly. Rarely, aggressive adenomas can invade the skull base.

Treatment is via surgical resection, usually from a trans-sphenoidal approach. Note the close relationship of the sella turcica and the sphenoid sinus on sagittal image (**107B**). Radiation therapy is occasionally used for residual portions of tumour that could not be safely resected (often within, or in close association with, the cavernous sinus).

TEACHING PEARLS
> ➤ *Pituitary macroadenomas measure greater than 1 cm by definition.*
> ➤ *These lesions generally come to medical attention due to mass effect upon, or invasion of, adjacent structures.*
> ➤ *Treatment is usually via trans-sphenoidal resection.*

REFERENCES
Jane JA, Laws ER (2003). The management of nonfunctioning pituitary adenomas. *Neurol India* **51**(4):461–5.
Kreutzer J, Fahlbusch R (2004). Diagnosis and treatment of pituitary tumours. *Curr Opin Neurol* **17**:693–703.

---

108 A 5-year-old female presents with nausea and vomiting, and the following images are obtained (**108A, B**).
i. Where is the mass located?
ii. What is the differential diagnosis?

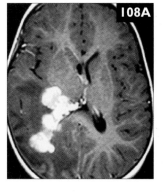
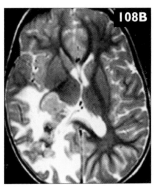

108 **DIAGNOSIS** Choroid plexus carcinoma.

IMAGING FINDINGS Images 108A, B (contrast-enhanced T1-weighted and T2-weighted MR images) demonstrate a strongly enhancing neoplasm of the atrium of the right lateral ventricle that extends into adjacent cerebral parenchyma, and is surrounded by marked oedema, mass effect, and left midline shift (i).

DIFFERENTIAL DIAGNOSIS The differential diagnosis of a trigonal lateral ventricular mass includes choroid plexus papilloma, choroid plexus carcinoma (rare), ependymoma, metastases, meningioma, and choroid plexus cyst (ii). The diagnosis is suggested in this case by the 'frond-like' appearance and parenchymal invasion – the later feature favouring choroid plexus carcinoma.

PATHOLOGY AND CLINICAL CORRELATION Choroid plexus carcinoma is an intraventricular lesion that occurs most commonly in the lateral ventricle. Although it can be difficult to differentiate from choroid plexus papilloma, the presence of parenchymal invasion is a more specific finding. Lesions occur before 5 years of age. On imaging, there is heterogeneous enhancement. Calcification is seen in a minority of cases. Screening of the entire neuraxis is crucial to evaluate for CSF dissemination.

TEACHING PEARLS
➤ *Imaging alone cannot reliably distinguish choroid plexus papilloma from carcinoma, although choroid plexus carcinoma is extremely rare. Definitive diagnosis is histological.*
➤ *Screening of the entire neuraxis for potential CSF dissemination is crucial.*

REFERENCES
Knierim DS, *et al.* (1991). Choroid plexus tumor in infants. *Pediatr Neurosurg* 16:276–80.
Osborn AG, *et al.* (2004). *Brain*. Amirsys, Salt Lake City, Chapter I-6, pp. 60–5.

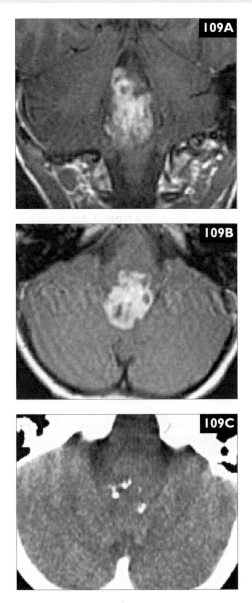

109 i. Where is this lesion located (**109A–C**)?
ii. Does the CT aid in the diagnosis in this case?

211

109 **DIAGNOSIS** Ependymoma.

IMAGING FINDINGS A heterogeneously enhancing neoplasm, arising from the floor of the 4th ventricle, is demonstrated in images **109A–C** (coronal T1 post-gadolinium, axial T1 post-gadolinium, and axial unenhanced CT). The mass expands the contour of the 4th ventricle, but without extension in this case into the foramen of Magendie. Several punctate foci of mineralization are noted within the mass on CT (**i, ii**).

DIFFERENTIAL DIAGNOSIS The broad differential diagnosis of a 4th ventricle mass includes ependymoma, choroid plexus papilloma/carcinoma, subependymoma, metastasis, atypical teratoid–rhabdoid tumour, or epidermoid tumour. Medulloblastoma (PNET), which strictly speaking does not arise from the ependymal lining of the ventricular system, but rather posterior to the 4th ventricular wall, can mimic an ependymoma, when large, by expanding into the 4th ventricle. Ependymal spread of tumour through the foramina of Luschka and/or Magendie is possible with true 4th ventricular masses such as ependymoma, but not with mimics such as medulloblastoma.

PATHOLOGY AND CLINICAL CORRELATION Ependymoma is the third most common paediatric posterior fossa lesion (after pilocytic astrocytoma and medulloblastoma). They characteristically expand to fill the 4th ventricle, and spread along the foramina of Luschka and Magendie into the cisterns. Lesions are may be infratentorial (4th ventricle) or supratentorial (periventricular). Calcification is common, as is haemorrhage. The typical patients is young (< 5 years old), and presents with signs and symptoms of hydrocephalus and increased intracranial pressure.

TEACHING PEARLS
- *Ependymoma is a lobular enhancing mass that can spread out the 4th ventricle through the foramen of Luschka (sometimes referred to as a 'toothpaste' or 'plastic' appearance).*
- *Ependymomas are often heterogenous, calcified and haemorrhagic; more so than medlulloblastomas.*
- *Sagittal imaging reveals the lesions origin at the floor of the 4th ventricle.*
- *Clinical profile: 1–5 year olds with headache and vomiting.*

REFERENCES
Osborn AG, *et al.* (2004) *Brain.* Amirsys, Salt Lake City, Chapter I-6, pp. 52–5.
Spoto GP, *et al.* (1990). Intracranial ependymoma and subependymoma: MR manifestations. *AJNR* 11:83–91.

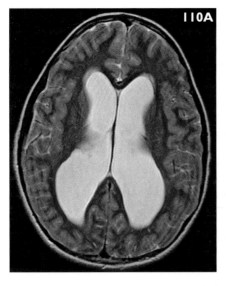

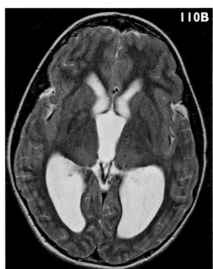

110 A child presents with morning headaches, and the following images are obtained (110A–C).

i. Is most hydrocephalus due to cerebrospinal fluid (CSF) overproduction, or to an obstruction preventing resorption of CSF?

ii. What are the two classic subtypes of obstructive hydrocephalus?

iii. Name several common symptoms of increased intracranial pressure.

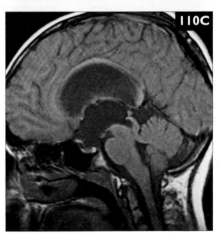

110 DIAGNOSIS Hydrocephalus.

IMAGING FINDINGS Note the marked dilatation of the lateral and 3rd ventricles on T2-weighted images (**110A, B**). Faint anterior periventricular parenchymal T2 hyperintensity is present. Sagittal T1 image (**110C**) confirms distention of the 3rd ventricle and demonstrates the 4th ventricle to be normal in size. In addition, there is apparent stenosis or occlusion of the aqueduct of Sylvius.

DIFFERENTIAL DIAGNOSIS When dilated ventricles are encountered, the primary distinction is between atrophy and hydrocephalus. A smooth border of increased T2 signal adjacent to the lateral ventricle lining due to transependymal resorption of CSF can be a clue that acute hydrocephalus is present. If there is no sulcal prominence to suggest diffuse atrophy, the general diagnosis of hydrocephalus is made. The next step in diagnosis is to further characterize the hydrocephalus as a sequela of increased CSF production (is there a choroid plexus papilloma?) or obstruction of CSF flow and resorption (the vast majority of cases) (i). In this case, as in most, we are dealing with the latter group.

The next step in the diagnostic process is to distinguish between the two subtypes of obstructive hydrocephalus, noncommunicating or communicating (ii). In noncommunicating hydrocephalus, there is a mechanical obstruction between the choroid plexus (where CSF is produced) and the outlet foramina of the 4th ventricle. Common sites include the foramen of Monro and the Sylvian aqueduct. In communicating hydrocephalus, the obstruction to CSF flow occurs more distally, most commonly at the arachnoid villi (where CSF is resorbed). Since there is ventricular dilatation only proximal to obstruction, the site of obstruction can usually be inferred by size evaluation of each ventricle separately. There is an extensive differential diagnosis for hydrocephalus based on the level of obstruction. In this case, the cause for the noncommunicating hydrocephalus can be identified as aqueductal stenosis.

PATHOLOGY AND CLINICAL CORRELATION Hydrocephalus is commonly encountered in neuroradiology and its complete understanding is often taken for granted. As noted above, this process is not a single pathologic entity but represents a shared common pathway of a diverse group of clinical scenarios, resulting in increased volume of CSF. Hydrocephalus is subdivided based on CSF overproduction or under-resorption.As less than 0.5% of cases are caused by CSF overproduction, the more useful distinction is between the subtypes of obstructive hydrocephalus, noncommunicating or communicating. Terminology in this regard is somewhat antiquated. As noted above, the arbitrary point of the outlet foramina of the fourth ventricle is the discriminator. Careful search for an obstructive lesion should always be undertaken and guided by the principle that obstruction should only cause proximal dilatation. Thus, dilation of all four ventricles usually implies communicating hydrocephalus. In this subset, a distinct lesion is usually not seen. Obstruction of the arachnoid villi is microscopic and commonly caused by blood products or protein from prior haemorrhage or infection.

Presentation is varied but symptoms generally relate to increased intracranial pressure. In adults, common signs include headache, nausea and vomiting, and are often most pronounced in the early morning hours (**iii**). In neonates and young children before the cranial sutures are fused, hydrocephalus often presents as increased head circumference. The increase in pressure can occur over varied time courses. A rapid rise in pressure can result in severe neurological compromise and even death.

TEACHING PEARLS
➤ *Hydrocephalus is a common pathway of multiple disorders rather than a single pathologic entity.*
➤ *Terminology is based on the mechanical cause of hydrocephalus and is most commonly (>99%) due to obstruction of CSF flow.*
➤ *Obstructive hydrocephalus is further divided into noncommunicating and communicating subtypes, based on location of obstruction proximal or distal to the outlet foramina of the 4th ventricle, respectively.*

REFERENCES
Bradley WG (2001). Diagnostic tools in hydrocephalus. *Neurosurg Clin N Am* **12**(4):661–84.
Pattisapu JV (2001). Etiology and clinical course of hydrocephalus. *Neurosurg Clin N Am* **12**(4):651–60.

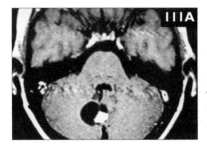 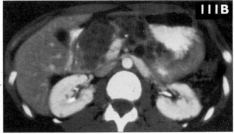

111 A 23-year-old female presents, receiving follow-up for a known condition, and the following images are obtained (**111A, B**). She reports that her mother, who died of renal cell carcinoma, had the same condition.
i. What is the differential diagnosis for the posterior fossa lesion?
ii. How does the abdominal CT help to narrow this differential diagnosis?

111 DIAGNOSIS Haemangioblastoma in von Hippel–Lindau (VHL) disease.

IMAGING FINDINGS Image **111A** shows a cystic appearing lesion with an intensely enhancing mural nodule that abuts the midline near the falx cerebelli. The axial abdominal CT image (**111B**) demonstrates a large cystic lesion of the pancreas and a possible mass within the medial right kidney.

DIFFERENTIAL DIAGNOSIS The differential diagnosis of a posterior fossa lesion in an adult includes metastases, haemangioblastoma, and astrocytoma (i). The appearance in this case is characteristic of haemangioblastoma. The appearance would also be similar to that of JPA, although this is less likely based on the abdominal CT findings.

PATHOLOGY AND CLINICAL CORRELATION Haemangioblastoma has a characteristic appearance of a cystic lesion with an intensely enhancing mural nodule abutting the pia, within the posterior fossa in an adult. Haemangioblastoma can also occur in the spinal cord and retina. VHL disease is an autosomal dominant condition characterized by haemangioblastomas and visceral cysts; various subtypes also include renal cell carcinoma and phaeochromocytoma. Multiple haemangioblastomas are diagnostic of VHL (ii), and screening of the entire CNS is required.

TEACHING PEARLS
➤ *Metastasis is the most common infratentorial neoplasm in adults. Approximately 25–40% of haemangioblastomas are associated with VHL.*
➤ *Haemangioblastoma classically presents as a cystic appearing lesion with enhancing mural nodule, abutting the pia mater in the posterior fossa, typically lateral to the 4th ventricle, and hence resembles JPA in children.*

REFERENCES
Conway JE, *et al.* (2001). Hemangioblastoma of the CNS in von Hippel–Lindau syndrome and sporadic disease. *Neurosurg* 48:55–63.
Osborn AG, *et al.* (2004). *Brain.* Amirsys, Salt Lake City, Chapter I-6, pp. 114–17.

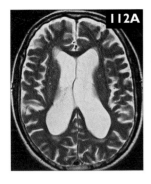
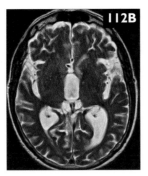
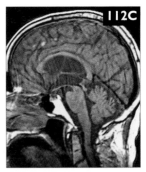

112 A patient presents with difficulty initiating walking, and the following images are obtained (112A–C).
i. Does the ventricular size correlate with the degree of peripheral cortical volume loss?
ii. What is the general pattern of hydrocephalus demonstrated?
iii. Where is the primary site of cerebrospinal fluid (CSF) resorption?

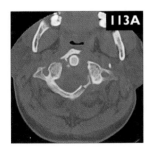
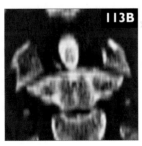
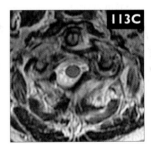

113 A 24-year-old patient presents after a multiple vehicle accident, and the following images are obtained (113A–C).
i. What is the name given to a C1 burst fracture affecting both the anterior and posterior arches?
ii. Is this a stable fracture?
iii. What is the most widely accepted model of thoracolumbar spinal trauma?

(The Answer to Case 113 is on page 220.)

112 **DIAGNOSIS** Normal pressure hydrocephalus (NPH).

IMAGING FINDINGS Axial T2 images demonstrate dilated lateral and 3rd ventricles (112A, B). Sagittal T1-weighted image confirms 3rd ventricular dilatation with superior bowing of the corpus callosum. No obstructing mass is present to account for the ventricular dilatation. Note the disproportionate ventricular prominence as compared to the relatively mild peripheral volume loss (i).

DIFFERENTIAL DIAGNOSIS The findings demonstrated are those of communicating hydrocephalus (ii). The actual diagnosis of NPH is clinical and, in addition to imaging findings of communicating hydrocephalus, requires normal CSF pressure and at least one finding of the classic NPH clinical triad (gait abnormality, urinary incontinence, and/or mental deficit). The primary differential consideration is volume loss/atrophy. The key to diagnosis of communicating hydrocephalus rather than atrophy is ventriculosulcal discordance. Ventricles are dilated 'out of proportion' to the degree of cortical volume loss and sulcal prominence. However, this can be a difficult distinction as there is often a degree of volume loss in patients with communicating hydrocephalus. Note that Sylvian fissures are also dilated in NPH.

PATHOLOGY AND CLINICAL CORRELATION NPH is a distinct entity that is not well understood. Since it was first described, the definition has been expanded and now includes most forms of chronic communicating hydrocephalus. As noted above, clinical diagnosis is based on imaging and physical findings. Radiological suggestion can be made when ventricular size is disproportionably large for the degree of sulcal prominence and patient history fits the clinical triad.

Though the aetiology of NPH is incompletely understood, the underlying abnormality appears to be decreased CSF resorption through the usual pathways at the arachnoid villi (iii). Approximately half of patients have a known cause for this lack of resorption (usually prior subarachnoid haemorrhage or meningitis), but the other half do not and are classified as 'idiopathic'. One theory to explain the many idiopathic cases is that the arachnoid villi are dysfunctional from birth in these patients, but CSF is resorbed through accessory parenchymal transvenous channels. As the patients age and develop microvascular disease, these accessory channels are damaged and can no longer handle the normal volume of resorption. This theory correlates well with the onset of disease. Patients with chronic communicating hydrocephalus from a known cause tend to present earlier, while those with the idiopathic form usually present with concordant microvascular disease after 60 years of age.

Regardless of the cause of communicating hydrocephalus, the next step in the evolution of the disease appears to be transient elevated ventricular pressures resulting in dilated lateral and 3rd ventricles. As the ventricular size increases, the pressure decreases to normal levels establishing a compensated form of communicating hydrocephalus with normal CSF pressure. Rather than eventually returning to normal ventricular size, these patients chronically maintain a dilated ventricular state. It has been postulated that this is due to an inherent abnormality in the viscoelastic properties of the affected parenchyma, eventually resulting in decreased compliance to CSF pulsation (generated by transmission from arterial blood flow). Since force is equal to pressure times area ($F = P \times A$), even with normal pressure, CSF pulsations exert an increased 'water hammer' force on the adjacent parenchyma due to markedly increased ventricular surface area. This primarily affects the periventricular neural tracts that supply the legs, accounting for the initial clinical sign of gait disturbance.

Treatment is variable. Some patients benefit from ventricular shunting. Several tests are used to determine which patients should benefit from this procedure. MRI findings that suggest hyperdynamic CSF pulsation are said to be a clue to shunt responsiveness. This is manifest by flow voids within the aqueduct and forth ventricle, seen best on proton density-weighted nonflow-compensated images. Some centres use the more specific quantitative phase contrast CSF velocity imaging to identify patients with elevated CSF flow though the cerebral aqueduct. The 'tap test' is often used clinically and consists of removing 50–60 cc of CSF and observing the patient. Those who then show a decrease in symptoms are good candidates for permanent shunt placement.

TEACHING PEARLS
➤ *NPH is a poorly understood form of compensated communicating hydrocephalus.*
➤ *The diagnosis of NPH is made clinically rather than through imaging.*
➤ *NPH is a form of potentially reversible dementia as some patients benefit from CSF shunting.*

REFERENCES
Bradley WG (2001). Diagnostic tools in hydrocephalus. *Neurosurg Clin N Am* **12**(4):661–84.

Hakim CA, Hakim RH, Hakim S (2001). Normal-pressure hydrocephalus. *Neurosurg Clin N Am* **12**(4):761–73.

Hurley RA, *et al.* (1999). Normal pressure hydrocephalus: significance of MRI in a potentially treatable dementia. *J Neuropsychiatry Clin Neurosci* **11**(3):297–300.

113 **Diagnosis** Jefferson fracture (C1 burst fracture).

Imaging findings There are at least three points of fracture involving both the anterior and posterior arches of the C1 ring apparent on this single axial CT image (**113A**). Coronal CT reformation (**113B**) confirms the lateral masses of C1 are displaced laterally as compared to the C2 lateral masses. Oblique, thin cut T2-weighted axial MRI image through the C1 level (**113C**) shows laxity of the transverse ligament indicating a tear (or avulsion) related to the fracture.

Differential diagnosis There is essentially no differential in this case of obvious fracture. It should be noted that ring structures such as the C1 vertebrae and all vertebral posterior elements generally fracture in at least two locations. When one fracture is identified, careful scrutiny should be given to the remainder of the ring.

Pathology and clinical correlation A complete discussion of spinal trauma/ fractures is well beyond the realm of this answer. However, several fundamental points are worthy of special emphasis. In general, spinal fractures can be divided into minor isolated posterior element fractures and more serious fractures involving the vertebral bodies. Vertebral body fractures are often discussed in terms of mechanism with flexion, extension, rotation, shear, and axial load providing the basic five forces of injury.

Within the upper cervical spine, several special types of the more common fractures deserve mention. Beginning superiorly, a Jefferson's fracture is an unstable fracture resulting from axial loading that involves multiple fracture points of the C1 ring, as in this case (**i,ii**). AP or open-mouth radiographs (and coronally reformatted CT) demonstrate lateral subluxation of the C1 lateral masses relative to C2. Another common cervical fracture involves the odontoid process (or dens) of C2. These fractures are classified based on the location of transverse fracture. Type I fractures involve only the tip of the dens. Type II fractures are the most common, are unstable, and traverse the base of the dens immediately superior to the C2 body. Type III fractures extend into the C2 body itself. A third type of common cervical fracture involves bilateral posterior elements at C2. This hyperextension injury is referred to as a hangman's fracture. Though most patients suffer no immediate neurological injury, this fracture is considered unstable.

The most widely accepted model of lower cervical and thoracolumbar fractures is the three-column model originally proposed in 1983 by Francis Denis (**iii**). This model defines the anterior column as composed of the anterior vertebral body, anterior longitudinal ligament, and anterior annulus fibrosus. The middle column consists of the posterior vertebral body wall, posterior longitudinal ligament, and posterior annulus fibrosus. The posterior column includes the posterior bony arch and associated ligamentous complex. In general, the number of columns affected in an injury correlates with the risk of neurological findings and potential for instability. Fractures (such as simple wedge compression fractures) that involve only the anterior column are considered stable. Two-column injuries are unstable or potentially unstable and three-column injuries are all considered extremely unstable. It appears that injuries involving the middle column are the most severe.

When related to the spinal column, it is important to realize that 'fractures' can involve either bone or soft tissue structures such as intervertebral discs or ligaments. While high resolution CT scan with sagittal and coronal reformatted images provide a great evaluation of bone, they often miss significant soft tissue injury. Therefore, complete spinal evaluation in a severe injury includes MRI (with STIR sequence) to better evaluate for soft tissue injury. Furthermore, associated spinal contusion, laceration, or epidural haematoma can also be readily identified with MRI. Countless studies have shown standard radiographs to be less sensitive for spinal injury than originally thought. Therefore, if there is any concern for significant injury, cross-sectional imaging is a must.

TEACHING PEARLS

➤ *The three-column model of spinal injury can be applied to the lower cervical, thoracic, and lumbar spine. Using this model, the number of columns affected correlates with the degree of instability and potential for neurological impairment.*

➤ *Radiographs alone can miss a significant number of spinal fractures. Cross-sectional imaging is recommended if significant injury is suspected.*

➤ *Spinal 'fractures' can involve both bone and soft tissue structures.*

REFERENCES

Denis F (1983). The three-column spine and its significance in classification of acute thoracolumbar spinal injuries. *Spine* 8(8):817–31.

Holmes JF, Akkinepalli R (2005). Computed tomography versus plain radiography to screen for cervical spine injury: a meta-analysis. *J Trauma* 58(5):902–5.

Osborn A (1994). *Diagnostic Neuroradiology*. Mosby, St Louis, pp. 20867–72.

Index